DRUG RESISTANT TUBERCULOSIS

Practical Guide for Clinical Management

Authored By

Rafael Laniado-Laborín

Clínica y Laboratorio de Tuberculosis

Hospital General Tijuana, México

DRUG RESISTANT TUBERCULOSIS

Bentham Science Publishers Ltd.
Executive Suite Y - 2
PO Box 7917, Saif Zone
Sharjah, U.A.E.
Email: subscriptions@benthamscience.org

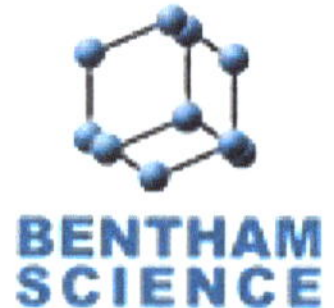

CONTENTS

FOREWORD

Drug-resistant tuberculosis (DR-TB) has become one of the main obstacles for global control of the disease. This problem, generated by inadequate treatment is particularly worrisome when resistance includes isoniazid (H) and rifampin (R) simultaneously, the most potent and active drugs against *Mycobacterium tuberculosis*. Treatment for this form of TB known as multidrug-resistant tuberculosis (MDR-TB) requires a minimum of 18-24 months of treatment with drugs that are less effective, more toxic and more expensive than those needed for drug-susceptible TB; unfortunately the rate of success of treatment for this form of TB hardly reach 70%.

As it is well known, prognosis of drug-resistant TB worsens even more when drug resistance extends to include fluoroquinolones and second-line injectables, the two most useful groups of the second-line drugs. This form of TB is known as extensive drug resistant TB or XDR-TB has even worst prognosis with a cure rate of only 50%.

Unfortunately, the extensive and inadequate use of rifampin in the past 30 years has generated an ever increasing number of MDR-TB cases that has reached epidemic levels in some regions of the world. It is estimated that by the year 2013 there were more than 480,000 cases of MDR-TB and that more than half of them were new cases never treated before, and thus the result of transmission of drug-resistant strains in the community and confirms its epidemic nature.

This growing scenario of MDR and XDR-TB has many experts considering that we are going to face soon forms of TB that will be virtually incurable. This, however, is not true since all forms of TB, even those with the most extensive degree of resistance have a possibility of being cured. This will depend decisively on the adequacy of the medical treatment available and this in turn will depend on the standards of quality for the programmatic management of TB by national TB programs.

For this reason, sound clinical management of patients with suspected or confirms DR-TB is fundamental for successful management. And here lies the problem, since DR-TB is a relatively recent phenomenon for which, the best clinical approach has not been fully standardized. Standardization of this complex clinical problem is therefore urgently needed. That is why, that books like this one, written in a rational and simple style by Dr. Laniado, are very helpful for clinicians caring for these unfortunate patients.

I was fortunate to meet Dr. Laniado in his native Tijuana, Mexico. And from the beginning I knew that I had the luck to become acquainted with a clinician that not only had exquisite knowledge of TB and MDR-TB, but also had the passion and dedication to his patients and the will to explore to the maximum their possibilities of being cured. During all these years, many patients have benefited from the quality and warmth that Dr. Laniado offers them every day. He has published extensively from his TB Clinic in Tijuana. And now we are in luck that he has dedicated innumerable hours to this book in which in a very straightforward way presents the fundamental principles of the best clinical management that can be offered to these patients. There will be many clinicians, pulmonologists and nonpulmonologists that will benefit from this nice treatise.

Jose A. Caminero
Coordinator, MDR-TB Unit
International Unit against Tuberculosis and Lung Diseases (The Union)
Paris, France
Servicio de Neumología
Hospital General de Gran Canaria "Dr. Negrin"
Las Palmas de Gran Canaria
España

"We have known how to cure TB for more than 50 years. What we have lacked is the will and the resources to quickly diagnose people with TB and get them the treatment they need."

Nelson Mandela, (1918-2013)

PREFACE

The emergence of highly drug-resistant strains of *Mycobacterium tuberculosis* (MTB) threatens to undermine global advances in tuberculosis (TB) control and challenges the goal of elimination of TB in the 21st century; unfortunately, despite rampant drug resistance in many regions of the world, TB is still extremely unpopular as a field of interest to clinicians, policymakers, and the media.

We have unfortunately witnessed an accelerated progression in resistance in many of the high TB-burden countries: multidrug-resistant TB being followed by extensively drug-resistant which in turn has been followed by what has been called totally drug-resistant TB which represents the most extreme form of amplified drug resistance.

The main objective of this practical guide is to help those physicians who are not experts in drug resistant tuberculosis but have to diagnose and treat such cases in everyday practice. It includes a description of the latest diagnostic tests and treatment regimens for the different types of drug-resistant tuberculosis. In the last chapter, we have included a series of hypothetical cases to illustrate some of the most frequent problems encountered while treating patients "in the real world". I sincerely hope that this work meets its goal.

Rafael Laniado-Laborín
Clínica y Laboratorio de Tuberculosis Hospital General Tijuana
México

CHAPTER 1

Epidemiology of Drug Resistant Tuberculosis

Abstract: In its Global Tuberculosis Report for 2013, the World Health Organization (WHO) estimated a total of 8.6 million tuberculosis (TB) incident cases and 1.3 million deaths from the disease during the previous year. Most of the drug resistant TB (DR-TB) cases were not even detected due to a variety of weaknesses of national TB programs. Only 28% of the 300,000 pulmonary TB patients expected to have MDR-TB in the world were reported; the WHO estimates that globally 3.6% of new TB cases and 20.2% of previously treated cases have MDR-TB, and of those, approximately 9.6% will have XDR-TB. In 2012 only 5% of the strains from new bacteriologically-confirmed TB cases and 9% of those previously treated for TB were cultured and tested for drug susceptibility. Outcome of treatment for patients with extensively drug resistance TB (XDR-TB) in a cohort from 26 countries was dismal with an overall cure rate of 20% and a 44% death rate.

Keywords: Bacteriological, Cohort, Countries, Death, DOT, Drug, Epidemiology, Global Report, MDR-TB, Pulmonary, Rates, Resistance, Self-administered, Tuberculosis, WHO, XDR-TB.

INTRODUCTION

The epidemic of drug resistance tuberculosis has evolved over the past 40 years, with resistance patterns progressively more complex and difficult to treat [1, 2].

In its Global Tuberculosis Report for 2013, the World Health Organization (WHO) [3] estimated a total of 8.6 million tuberculosis (TB) incident cases and 1.3 million deaths from the disease in 2012. Most of the drug resistant TB (DR-TB) cases are not even detected due to a variety of weaknesses of national TB programs (lack of access to medical care, lack of laboratory support, insufficient drugs supply, *etc.*).

Globally, only 28% of the estimated 300,000 MDR-TB cases were reported [3]. The WHO estimates that 3.6% of newly diagnosed TB cases and 20.2% of previously treated cases will have MDR-TB; of those an estimated 9.6% will have

Rafael Laniado-Laborín

XDR-TB, and according to that 2013 report, at least one case of XDR-TB has been reported in 92 countries. In 2012 only 5% of the strains from new bacteriologically-confirmed TB cases and 9% of those previously treated for TB were cultured and tested for drug susceptibility (DST) [3]. Reaching the WHO proposed goals of performing DST in at least 20% of new cases and in 100% of previously treated cases will be extremely difficult, since the countries with the highest burden of disease are those with the lowest income, with limited or no available laboratory facilities with the infrastructure needed for DR-TB diagnosis.

Drug susceptible TB has an expected cure rate of ≥95%; outcomes of treatment for patients with drug resistance are much lower. Globally, rates of success for treatment of MDR-TB are barely around 70%. Cure rate for extensively drug resistance TB (XDR-TB) in a 2012 cohort from 26 countries was even worst with an overall cure rate of 20% and a 44% death rate [3].

The heart of the WHO DOTS strategy is the directly observed treatment (DOT) component to guarantee adequate adherence, and although a recent meta-analysis [4] reported no statistical differences in rates of treatment failure, clinical relapse or acquired drug resistance between DOT and self-administered regimens (SAT), there might be concealed bias in the estimates, since patients are reported by TB programs frequently as in DOT when in reality they are under SAT [5].

CONFLICT OF INTEREST

The author confirms that this chapter has no conflict of interest.

ACKNOWLEDGEMENTS

None declared.

REFERENCES

[1] Migliori GB, Sotgiu G, D'Ambrosio L, *et al.* TB and MDR/XDR-TB in European Union and European Economic Area countries: managed or mismanaged? Eur Respir J 2012; 39(3): 619-25. [http://dx.doi.org/10.1183/09031936.00170411] [PMID: 22323578]

[2] Gandhi NR, Nunn P, Dheda K, *et al.* Multidrug-resistant and extensively drug-resistant tuberculosis: a threat to global control of tuberculosis. Lancet 2010; 375(9728): 1830-43. [http://dx.doi.org/10.1016/S0140-6736(10)60410-2] [PMID: 20488523]

[3] WHO Global Tuberculosis Report WHO/HTM/TB/ 2013; 11

[4] Pasipanodya JG, Gumbo T. A meta-analysis of self-administered *vs.* directly observed therapy effect on microbiologic failure, relapse, and acquired drug resistance in tuberculosis patients. Clin Infect Dis 2013; 57(1): 21-31.
[http://dx.doi.org/10.1093/cid/cit167] [PMID: 23487389]

[5] Radilla-Chávez P, Laniado-Laborín R. Results of directly observed treatment for tuberculosis in Ensenada, Mexico: not all DOTS programs are created equally. Int J Tuberc Lung Dis 2007; 11(3): 289-92.
[PMID: 17352094]

CHAPTER 2

Mycobacterium Tuberculosis: Etiological Agent of Tuberculosis

Abstract: The *Mycobacteria* genus, member of the *Mycobacteriacea* family and *Actinomycetales* order, are nonmotile, nonsporulating, acid-fast bacilli, 2-4 μ in length and 0.2-0.5 μ in width. Their waxy cell wall, rich in mycolic acid plays an important role in its resistance to many antibiotics. The *Mycobacterium genus* can be separated into two major groups. One group includes the *Mycobacterium tuberculosis* complex and the other includes non-tuberculous (also known as environmental) mycobacteria. The *Mycobacterium tuberculosis* complex includes *M. tuberculosis (Mtb), M. canettii, M. africanum, M. microti, M. bovis*, *M.caprae* and *M. pinnipedii*. Mycobacteria are facultative intracellular bacteria that multiply within phagocytic cells. In addition to the ability to acquire new resistance through the acquisition of chromosomal mutations, *Mtb* has a variety of intrinsic resistance mechanisms that allow active neutralization of antibiotic actions. *Mtb* intrinsic drug resistance can be divided into two categories: passive resistance and specialized resistance mechanisms; besides the cell wall barrier that helps slow down the penetration of antibiotics, *Mtb* operates multiple specialized resistance mechanisms that allow active detoxification of drugs once they reach the cytoplasmic space. *Mtb*, acquired drug resistance is caused by spontaneous random mutations in chromosomal genes, facilitating the selection of resistant strains during sub-optimal drug therapy. Clinically, drug resistance in *Mtb* represents the selection of random genetic mutations, not a change caused by exposure to the medication.

Keywords: Acquired resistance, Actinomicetales, Chromosome, Detoxification, Genus, Intrinsic resistance, *M. africanum*, *M. bovis*, *M. canettii*, *M.caprae* and *M. pinnipedii*, *M. microti*, *M. tuberculosis*, Mutations, Mycobacteria.

INTRODUCTION

The *Mycobacteria genus*, member of the *Mycobacteriacea* family and *Actinomycetales* order, are nonmotile, nonsporulating, acid-fast bacilli, 2-4 μ in length and 0.2-0.5 μ in width. Their waxy cell wall, rich in mycolic acid plays and is responsible for many of its biological characteristics: acid-fastness, variable degrees of hydrophobicity, resistance to drying, extreme changes in pH, and very

Rafael Laniado-Laborín

important from a clinical point of view, at least in part, resistance to many antibiotics [1]. Both acid-fastness and low permeability are due to the presence of long chain α-alkyl, β-hydroxy fatty acids in the cell wall [2].

The *Mycobacterium genus* can be separated into two major groups on the basis of their growth rate in solid cultures. One group includes slow-growing species: *Mycobacterium tuberculosis* complex, *Mycobacterium bovis* and *Mycobacterium leprae* (etiological agents of human tuberculosis, bovine tuberculosis and leprosy respectively); the other group includes fast-growing species such as *M. fortuitum* and *M. chelonae/abscessus*. The *Mycobacterium tuberculosis* complex refers to a group of species (*M. tuberculosis (Mtb), M. canettii, M. africanum, M. microti, M. bovis*, *M.caprae* and *M. pinnipedii*) that are genetically very similar. Although many mycobacterial species are environmental, *Mtb* is strictly parasitic and infects more than one-third of the world's human population. *M. canettii* and *M. africanum*, closely related to *Mtb*, can also cause human tuberculosis. In most cases reported in the literature this species has been isolated from African patients. *M. bovis* can infect humans, domestic or wild bovines and goats. Humans will usually acquire the infection by consumption of unpasteurized milk or unpasteurized milk products (*e.g.* fresh cheese). *M. caprae* has been isolated only from goats. *M. microti* is a rodent pathogen, usually isolated from voles that can also cause disease in immunocompromised human patients. Finally, *M. pinnipedii* infects seals [2].

As mentioned, *Mycobacterium tuberculosis* (*Mtb*) is a member of the *Mycobacterium tuberculosis* complex, characterized by a 24-36-hour division rate and prolonged culture period in solid media (4-8 weeks). As mentioned mycobacteria are facultative intracellular bacteria that multiply within phagocytic cells. If environmental conditions requires it, *Mtb* metabolism mode can change from an aerobic mode that obtains most of its energy from carbohydrates, to one with reduced oxygen requirements, obtaining most of its energy requirements from lipid substrates. When cultured in solid media (either Middlebrook's 7H10 agar medium or Lowenstein-Jensen egg based medium) *Mtb* colonies are small and beige colored [1, 2].

Basic Mechanisms of Drug resistance in *Mycobacterium Tuberculosis*

Although even wild strains of *Mycobacterium tuberculosis* will have some drug resistant bacteria as a result of spontaneous random mutations, the proportion in a given population of bacteria is so low (<1%) that this resistance is not clinically relevant. Significant drug resistance in TB, in the clinical setting is defined as the genetically increased capacity to survive and multiply when exposed to a specific drug (or drugs) in comparison to drug-susceptible bacillβ [3]. Furthermore, in addition to the ability to acquire new resistance through genetic mutations, *Mtb* has a variety of biological resistance mechanisms that allow active neutralization of antibiotic actions.

Mtb intrinsic drug resistance can be divided into two categories: passive resistance and specialized resistance mechanisms [4].

Passive Resistance Mechanisms

Mtb cell wall plays an important role in mycobacterial physical resistance mechanisms against antibiotics, limiting the degree of penetration of some of the antituberculosis drugs. Mycobacterial cell wall is thick, multi-layered and hydrophobic, preventing the transport of hydrophobic molecules, including antibiotics. Nonetheless, due to the prolonged doubling time of *Mtb* (24-36 hrs.), even the slow penetration rate of some antibiotics might in some cases be high enough to allow drugs to accumulate to inhibitory levels before cell division occurs [3 - 5].

Efflux mechanisms (mechanisms that transport compounds out of the cell) have also been recognized as an important factor in physical resistance of drug resistance in mycobacteria. Efflux pumps are physiologic mechanisms of mycobacteria for transportation of nutrients, toxins and waste through the cell wall. These mechanisms have evolved in mycobacteria and can also expel antibiotics using efflux pumps, including fluoroquinolones and aminoglycosides, among others [4].

Mycobacterium tuberculosis in most cases of human infection is inhaled to the lungs. *Mtb* are then phagocyted by alveolar macrophages and contained in phagosomes. Under normal circumstances, intracellular bacteria are destroyed when exposed to lysosomal enzymes; however, *Mtb* have developed a number of biological resistance mechanisms such as the inhibition of the phagosome-lysosome fusion, evading the lethal low pH inside the phagolysosome. In the immunocompetent host, infection by *Mtb* is usually contained in the lung through the formation of granulomas where some of the bacteria may remain dormant for years without active clinical disease (clinically known as latent tuberculosis). If the individual becomes immuno-compromised, latent bacteria can become active, with the development of clinical tuberculosis [2].

Specialized Resistance Mechanisms

Besides the cell wall barrier that helps slow down the penetration of antibiotics, *Mtb* operates multiple specialized resistance mechanisms that allow active detoxification of drugs once they reach the cytoplasmic space.

Mycobacteria can neutralize antibiotics through direct chemical modifications; for example, the metabolic pathway of acetylation is a vital process for mycobacterial resistance to aminoglycosides. Studies have identified homologs of aminoglycoside 2'- N-acetyltransferase (aac) in mycobacteria that confer resistance to amino-glucósidos [4 - 6].

Another pathway that *Mtb* uses to inactivate antibiotics is to directly degrade those using hydrolases. This mechanism is best studied in the case of β-lactams. These antibiotics inhibit cell wall biosynthesis, leading to cell death [4, 7]. Mycobacterial β-lactamases are generally less active than those of other pathogenic bacteria. However, due to the slow penetration of β-lactams across the thick cell wall of mycobacteria β-lactamase activity is effective enough to protect mycobacteria from β-lactam action. The most important β-lactamase in *Mtb* is BlaC, active against carbapenems, which arc generally resistant to β-lactamases of other pathogenic bacteria [8]. Besides BlaC, *Mtb* encodes at least three more β-lactamase genes: blaS, rv0406c and rv3677c [9]. The use of β-lactamase-resistant antibiotics or the combination of a β-lactam antibiotic plus a β-lactamase inhibitor has been shown to be effective in clinical settings [10, 11].

Mycobacteria can also neutralize antibiotics through molecular mimicry.

Fluoroquinolones, the most important class of antibiotics for the treatment of multidrug resistant TB, are bactericidal drugs that inhibit bacterial DNA replication, transcription and repair through their interaction with DNA gyrase; DNA degradation leads subsequently to cell death [3]. Mycobacteria have a protein (*MfpA*) that confers resistance to fluoroquinolones. The chemical structure of *MfpA* resembles the spatial structure of the bacterial DNA double helix [12]· The interaction between *MfpA* and the fluoroquinolones in the cytoplasm would protect the real DNA from the drug action [13].

Genetic Mechanisms of Drug Resistance in *Mycobacterium Tuberculosis*

The deciphering of the complete genome sequence of *Mtb* has established that specific gene mutations in mycobacteria are associated with very specific drug resistance (Table **2.1**) [14].

Table 2.1. Genes responsibly of acquired resistance in *M. tuberculosis*.

	Drug	Mode of action	Gene	Gene function
	Isoniazid	Inhibition of mycolic acid synthesis	*katG*	Catalase-peroxidase
			inhA	Enoyl ACP reductase
			inhA promoter	Regulation of expression of inhA
			ndh	NADH dehydrogenase II
First-line			*ahpC*	Alkyl hydroperoxidase
			fabG	3-oxoacyl-lthioester reductase
			fadE24	Fatty acid β-oxidation
			rpoA	α-subunit of RNA polymerase
	Rifampin	Inhibition of transcription	*rpoB*	β-subunit of RNA polymerase
			rpoC	β-subunit of RNA polymerase
	Pyrazinamide	Inhibition of trans-translation	*pncA*	Pyrazinamidase
			rspA	SI ribosomal protein
	Ethambutol	Inhibition of arabinogalactan sysnthesis	*embCAB*	Arabinosyltransferases
			embR	*emb* CAB transcription regulator

(Table 2.1) contd.....

	Streptomycin	Inhibition of translation	*rpsL*	S12 ribosomal protein
			rrs	16S sRNA
			gidB	16S sRNA methyltransferase
	Amikacin & Kanamycin	Inhibition of translation	*rrs*	16S sRNA
			eis	Acetyltransferase
	Capreomycin & viomycin	Alteration of drug target	*tlyA*	rRNA methyltransferase
			rrs	16S sRNA
Second-line	Ethionamide	Inhibition of mycolic acid synthesis	*inhA*	Enoyl ACP reductase
			inhA promoter	Regulation of expression of inhA
	Para-amino salicylic acid	Targeting DHFR	*thyA*	Thymidylate synthase A

The *Mtb* H37Rv genome consists of 4.4 A- 10^6 bp and contains approximately 4,000 genes. More than 200 genes have been classified as gene that encode enzymes involved in the metabolism of fatty acids. This large number of *Mtb* enzymes involved in lipids metabolism may explain the ability of *Mtb* to grow in tissues of the infected host where fatty acids may be the major energy source [15].

Unlike other type of bacteria, where acquired drug resistance is generally mediated through horizontal transfer of mobile genetic elements (*e.g.* plasmids) from one resistant bacteria to another previously susceptible bacteria, *Mtb*, acquired drug resistance is caused by spontaneous random mutations in chromosomal genes, facilitating the selection of resistant strains during sub-optimal drug therapy [14]. These mutations are unlinked; consequently, resistance to one class of drug is generally not associated with resistance to an ***unrelated*** class of drug (*e.g.* a mutation conferring resistance to a fluoroquinolone will not confer resistance to an aminoglycoside). The development of drug resistance represents the selection by inadequate treatment of random genetic mutations, not a transformation caused by exposure to antituberculosis drugs [16]. The rate of mutations conferring resistance in *Mtb* for most of the antituberculosis drugs occurs at a rate of between 10^8-10^9 mutations. The probability of a strain of *Mtb* being spontaneously resistant to isoniazid and rifampin would be equal to the product of their individual probabilities or 10^{16-18} . Noteven patients with extensive pulmonary disease harbor such large number of mycobacteria. Therefore, almost without exception a polyresistant, MDR or XDR *Mtb* strain will be man-made, the result of one or more inadequate treatment regimens.

Even though latent bacilli have a very slow rate of replication (with periods of non-replication) it has been reported that *Mtb* in latent status can mutate, and this spontaneous random mutations can result in drug resistance [17]. Some strains of *Mtb* seem to have higher mutation rates (and higher probability of acquiring resistance); it has been hypothesized that these strains have a "omutator genotype" [18]. An example of this would be a particular phylogenetic lineage of mycobacteria classified as the "*Beijing family*" that has been frequently associated with MDR-TB [19, 20].

Fitness Cost and Compensatory Mechanisms

How significantly drug resistant strains will influence the global TB epidemic will depend largely on their virulence when comparing it to drug-susceptible mycobacteria. Studies on the community transmission of TB have shown that MDR-TB strains differ on their transmission potential [19 - 21].

Old animal experiments from the 1950A's, reported that isoniazid-resistant *Mtb* strains were less virulent than drug susceptible *Mtb* [22]. These reports created the myth that drug-resistant *Mtb* were less virulent (less "biologically fit") and therefore less transmissible and unable to disseminate successfully in the community [23]. The hypothesis was that these mutations would affect mycobacterial fitness and their ability to spread in the community. However, this theoretical model has been proven wrong by several outbreaks of MDR-TB [3, 24]. This might explained by a phenomenon known as epistasis that is defined as the resulting effect of the interaction between two (or more) mutations of the mycobacterial phenotype, one conferring resistance to a drug and the other a compensatory mutation [25 - 29].

Drug resistant strains will only become predominant in *Mtb* populations if the resistance phenotypes provide the mutants with survival advantages over their susceptible counterparts. Poorly structured TB programs that lack adequate resources for directly observed therapy favor the steady evolution of *Mtb* strains that are progressively resistant to the available drugs. There is an increased probability that exposure of mycobacteria to inadequate levels of bactericidal drugs leads to increased mutations in other drug resistance genes [3, 30].

Another factor that contributes to antibiotic resistance is the dormant state that *Mtb* will display during latent infection, a state characterized by virtual shutdown of all metabolic functions [31]; drug resistance in these mycobacteria (also known as persisters) is due to its low metabolic rates rather than due to resistance mutations [32].

CONFLICT OF INTEREST

The author confirms that this chapter has no conflict of interest.

ACKNOWLEDGEMENTS

None declared.

REFERENCES

[1] Sakamoto K. The pathology of *Mycobacterium tuberculosis* infection. Vet Pathol 2012; 49(3): 423-39. [http://dx.doi.org/10.1177/0300985811429313] [PMID: 22262351]

[2] Forrellad MA, Klepp LI, GioffrA(c) A, *et al.* Virulence factors of the *Mycobacterium tuberculosis* complex. Virulence 2013; 4(1): 3-66. [http://dx.doi.org/10.4161/viru.22329] [PMID: 23076359]

[3] MA1/4ller B, Borrell S, Rose G, Gagneux S. The heterogeneous evolution of multidrug-resistant *Mycobacterium tuberculosis*. Trends Genet 2013; 29(3): 160-9. [http://dx.doi.org/10.1016/j.tig.2012.11.005] [PMID: 23245857]

[4] Smith T, Wolff KA, Nguyen L. Molecular biology of drug resistance in *Mycobacterium tuberculosis*. Curr Top Microbiol Immunol 2013; 374: 53-80. [http://dx.doi.org/10.1007/82_2012_279] [PMID: 23179675]

[5] Russell DG. The evolutionary pressures that have molded *Mycobacterium tuberculosis* into an infectious adjuvant. Curr Opin Microbiol 2013; 16(1): 78-84. [http://dx.doi.org/10.1016/j.mib.2012.11.007] [PMID: 23290190]

[6] Zaunbrecher MA, Sikes RD Jr, Metchock B, Shinnick TM, Posey JE. Overexpression of the chromosomally encoded aminoglycoside acetyltransferase eis confers kanamycin resistance in *Mycobacterium tuberculosis*. Proc Natl Acad Sci USA 2009; 106(47): 20004-9. [http://dx.doi.org/10.1073/pnas.0907925106] [PMID: 19906990]

[7] Chambers HF, Moreau D, Yajko D, *et al.* Can penicillins and other beta-lactam antibiotics be used to

treat tuberculosis? Antimicrob Agents Chemother 1995; 39(12): 2620-4.
[http://dx.doi.org/10.1128/AAC.39.12.2620] [PMID: 8592990]

[8] Hugonnet JE, Blanchard JS. Irreversible inhibition of the *Mycobacterium tuberculosis* beta-lactamase by clavulanate. Biochemistry 2007; 46(43): 11998-2004.
[http://dx.doi.org/10.1021/bi701506h] [PMID: 17915954]

[9] Flores AR, Parsons LM, Pavelka MS Jr. Genetic analysis of the beta-lactamases of *Mycobacterium tuberculosis* and *Mycobacterium smegmatis* and susceptibility to beta-lactam antibiotics. Microbiology 2005; 151(Pt 2): 521-32.
[http://dx.doi.org/10.1099/mic.0.27629-0] [PMID: 15699201]

[10] Voladri RK, Lakey DL, Hennigan SH, Menzies BE, Edwards KM, Kernodle DS. Recombinant expression and characterization of the major β-lactamase of *Mycobacterium tuberculosis*. Antimicrob Agents Chemother 1998; 42(6): 1375-81.
[PMID: 9624479]

[11] Hugonnet JE, Tremblay LW, Boshoff HI, Barry CE III, Blanchard JS. Meropenem-clavulanate is effective against extensively drug-resistant *Mycobacterium tuberculosis*. Science 2009; 323(5918): 1215-8.
[http://dx.doi.org/10.1126/science.1167498] [PMID: 19251630]

[12] Hegde SS, Vetting MW, Roderick SL, *et al.* A fluoroquinolone resistance protein from *Mycobacterium tuberculosis* that mimics DNA. Science 2005; 308(5727): 1480-3.
[http://dx.doi.org/10.1126/science.1110699] [PMID: 15933203]

[13] Ferber D. Biochemistry. Protein that mimics DNA helps tuberculosis bacteria resist antibiotics. Science 2005; 308(5727): 1393.
[http://dx.doi.org/10.1126/science.308.5727.1393a] [PMID: 15933168]

[14] Almeida Da Silva PE, Palomino JC. Molecular basis and mechanisms of drug resistance in *Mycobacterium tuberculosis*: classical and new drugs. J Antimicrob Chemother 2011; 66(7): 1417-30.
[http://dx.doi.org/10.1093/jac/dkr173] [PMID: 21558086]

[15] Smith I. *Mycobacterium tuberculosis* pathogenesis and molecular determinants of virulence. Clin Microbiol Rev 2003; 16(3): 463-96.
[http://dx.doi.org/10.1128/CMR.16.3.463-496.2003] [PMID: 12857778]

[16] Iseman MD. Treatment of multidrug-resistant tuberculosis. N Engl J Med 1993; 329(11): 784-91.
[http://dx.doi.org/10.1056/NEJM199309093291108] [PMID: 8350889]

[17] Ford CB, Lin PL, Chase MR, *et al.* Use of whole genome sequencing to estimate the mutation rate of *Mycobacterium tuberculosis* during latent infection. Nat Genet 2011; 43(5): 482-6.
[http://dx.doi.org/10.1038/ng.811] [PMID: 21516081]

[18] Jolivet-Gougeon A, Kovacs B, Le Gall-David S, *et al.* Bacterial hypermutation: clinical implications. J Med Microbiol 2011; 60(Pt 5): 563-73.
[http://dx.doi.org/10.1099/jmm.0.024083-0] [PMID: 21349992]

[19] Borrell S, Gagneux S. Infectiousness, reproductive fitness and evolution of drug-resistant *Mycobacterium tuberculosis*. Int J Tuberc Lung Dis 2009; 13(12): 1456-66.
[PMID: 19919762]

[20] Ebrahimi-Rad M, Bifani P, Martin C, *et al.* Mutations in putative mutator genes of *Mycobacterium tuberculosis* strains of the W-Beijing family. Emerg Infect Dis 2003; 9(7): 838-45. [http://dx.doi.org/10.3201/eid0907.020803] [PMID: 12890325]

[21] Brites D, Gagneux S. Old and new selective pressures on *Mycobacterium tuberculosis*. Infect Genet Evol 2012; 12(4): 678-85. [http://dx.doi.org/10.1016/j.meegid.2011.08.010] [PMID: 21867778]

[22] Barnett M, Busby SR, Mitchison DA. Tubercle bacillβresistant to isoniazid: virulence and response to treatment with isoniazid in guinea-pigs and mice. Br J Exp Pathol 1953; 34(5): 568-81. [PMID: 13106225]

[23] Keshavjee S, Farmer PE. Tuberculosis, drug resistance, and the history of modern medicine. N Engl J Med 2012; 367(10): 931-6. [http://dx.doi.org/10.1056/NEJMra1205429] [PMID: 22931261]

[24] Zignol M, van Gemert W, Falzon D, *et al.* Surveillance of anti-tuberculosis drug resistance in the world: an updated analysis, 2007-2010. Bull World Health Organ 2012; 90(2): 111-119D. [http://dx.doi.org/10.2471/BLT.11.092585] [PMID: 22423162]

[25] Phillips PC. Epistasis--the essential role of gene interactions in the structure and evolution of genetic systems. Nat Rev Genet 2008; 9(11): 855-67. [http://dx.doi.org/10.1038/nrg2452] [PMID: 18852697]

[26] Weinreich DM, Watson RA, Chao L. Perspective: Sign epistasis and genetic constraint on evolutionary trajectories. Evolution 2005; 59(6): 1165-74. [PMID: 16050094]

[27] Gagneux S, Long CD, Small PM, Van T, Schoolnik GK, Bohannan BJ. The competitive cost of antibiotic resistance in *Mycobacterium tuberculosis*. Science 2006; 312(5782): 1944-6. [http://dx.doi.org/10.1126/science.1124410] [PMID: 16809538]

[28] Billington OJ, McHugh TD, Gillespie SH. Physiological cost of rifampin resistance induced *in vitro* in *Mycobacterium tuberculosis*. Antimicrob Agents Chemother 1999; 43(8): 1866-9. [PMID: 10428904]

[29] Mariam DH, Mengistu Y, Hoffner SE, Andersson DI. Effect of rpoB mutations conferring rifampin resistance on fitness of *Mycobacterium tuberculosis*. Antimicrob Agents Chemother 2004; 48(4): 1289-94. [http://dx.doi.org/10.1128/AAC.48.4.1289-1294.2004] [PMID: 15047531]

[30] Kohanski MA, Dwyer DJ, Collins JJ. How antibiotics kill bacteria: from targets to networks. Nat Rev Microbiol 2010; 8(6): 423-35. [http://dx.doi.org/10.1038/nrmicro2333] [PMID: 20440275]

[31] Gengenbacher M, Kaufmann SH. *Mycobacterium tuberculosis*: success through dormancy. FEMS Microbiol Rev 2012; 36(3): 514-32. [http://dx.doi.org/10.1111/j.1574-6976.2012.00331.x] [PMID: 22320122]

[32] Garton NJ, Waddell SJ, Sherratt AL, *et al.* Cytological and transcript analyses reveal fat and lazy persister-like bacilli in tuberculous sputum. PLoS Med 2008; 5(4): e75. [http://dx.doi.org/10.1371/journal.pmed.0050075] [PMID: 18384229]

CHAPTER 3

Biological Basis for Drug Resistant Tuberculosis

Abstract: This chapter deals with the classification and mechanisms of drug resistance in tuberculosis, from mono-resistant to extensive drug resistance (XDR) strains. Resistance can be classified as "new cases" for patients never treated before (or treated for less than a month) with antituberculosis drugs and infected by an already drug resistant strain, and "previously treated cases". There are multiple factors associated to drug resistance but they can be grouped in three basic categories: clinical, biological and social factors. Clinical factors include, among others, inadequate treatment regimens (wrong drugs, wrong doses), using drugs of unproven quality, drug shortages, and treatment with weak regimens by private physicians. Biological factors can include factors both the host and from the mycobacteria: being infected with an already resistant strain or host immunosuppression. Social factors include residing in areas with high rates of DR-TB, extreme poverty and lack of social support, illiteracy, poorly structured and supported TB control programs and lack of political compromise.

Keywords: AIDS, Beijing, Extensive drug resistance, HIV, Immunosuppression, MDR, Mono-resistance. poly-resistance, Multidrug resistant, Mycobacteria, Susceptible, Virulent, XDR.

INTRODUCTION

Definition and Classification of Drug Resistance to Antituberculosis Drugs

Drug resistance to antituberculosis drugs is defined as [1]:

a. Mono-resistance: resistance to one antituberculosis drug
b. Poly-resistance: resistance to two or more antituberculosis drugs that are not isoniazid and rifampin simultaneously
c. Multidrug resistance (MDR-TB): simultaneous resistance to at least isoniazid and rifampin simultaneously
d. XDR TB: extensively resistant strains that are resistant to at least isoniazid and rifampin from the first line drugs, plus resistant to any fluoroquinolone and at least to one of the second line injectables (kanamycin, amikacin, capreomycin)

Rafael Laniado-Laborín

e. Resistance greater than XDR: also known as totally resistant TB (TDR-TB); it refers to resistance to all 12 traditional antituberculosis drugs

Resistance can also be classified as "new cases" for patients never treated before (or treated for less than a month) with antituberculosis drugs and infected by an already drug resistant strain, and "previously treated cases".

Treatment strategies for tuberculosis are very different from those used in other bacterial infections. *M. tuberculosis* has a very prolonged generation time (>24 hours); it has also the ability to adopt a latent status with virtual shutdown of all metabolic activity making it a difficult target for most therapeutic agents. *Mtb* thrives in lung cavities and even survives in necrotic areas, sites where penetration of antibiotics is low and where the acidic tissue pH inhibits most antimicrobials including the antituberculosis injectables (pyrazinamide on the other hand is highly active in the acidic intracellular environment). Concentrations of mycobacteria will vary within a host depending on the site: mycobacteria will rapidly multiply on the oxygen-rich lung cavities, while they will adopt a latent status, multiplying only occasionally within necrotic foci [2].

Factors Associated to The Development of Drug Resistance

There are multiple factors associated to drug resistance but they can be group in three basic categories: clinical, biological and social factors.

Clinical factors include, among others, inadequate treatment regimens (wrong drugs, wrong doses), using drugs of unproven quality, drug shortages, treatment with weak regimens by private physicians.

Biological factors can include factors both the host and from the mycobacteria: being infected with an already resistant strain (new case DR-TB), highly resistant strains (Beijing or "W") or host immunosuppression (HIV, malnutrition, diabetes, *etc.*)

Social factors are very important in the genesis of DR-TB and include residing in areas with high rates of DR-TB, extreme poverty and lack of social support, illiteracy, lack of adherence to treatment regimen, poorly structured and supported TB control programs and lack of political compromise [3].

Prescription of inadequate drug regimens is one of the major culprits involved in the development of DR-TB. A poorly structured (and supported) TB control program will create more drug resistant cases than those that it will be able to treat. This is due to lack of directly observed therapy and poor adherence of self administered treatment, use of drugs of poor quality, treatment of relapses, failures and defaulters with first line drugs without the benefit of DST to determine the presence or absence of drug resistance. Under these conditions, a progressively greater proportion of TB cases will be caused by drug resistant strains. When a TB program is unable to diagnose and treat DR cases, it will only cure drug susceptible cases (and with a lower rate of success than expected due to the conditions just mentioned) and drug resistant cases will be gradually selected. The vast majority of drug resistant cases are cases that have been previously inadequately treated (less than 4% of global MDR-TB cases are new cases) [2].

There are several factors that contribute to the selection of mutant resistant strains in patients previously treated for tuberculosis; these include treatment default associated to intolerance of drug regimen due to side effects and/or toxicity, disbelief of the diagnosis or necessity of treatment, alcohol or drug abuse and neuropsychiatric disease [4].

It is well known that not every subject infected with *Mtb* will develop active disease. Approximately 10% of infected individuals without immunosuppressive diseases will eventually develop clinical active disease, most within 18 months of being infected. However, even with this scenario, in communities with high rates of drug-resistant TB, a substantial proportion of that 10% will have a resistant strain as a causative agent. As mentioned in chapter 2, the time-honored idea that drug resistant *Mtb* strains are less virulent than drug susceptible mycobacteria has been proven wrong by the numerous outbreaks of DR-TB reported in the literature [5].

The Human Immunodeficiency Virus (HIV) epidemic has affected mainly those population groups that have also high rates of tuberculosis (particularly due to the fact that both diseases share a common risk factor which is poverty). Since HIV infection affects cellular immunity, the most vital element of the immune response to tuberculosis infection, the AIDS epidemic has created a dramatic global resurgence of tuberculosis. An extraordinarily alarming aspect of this epidemic is the increasing rates of XDR-TB in individuals co-infected with HIV in some regions of the world [6]. The outbreaks of DR-TB in Sub-Saharan Africa are a catastrophic example of this phenomenon [7].

CONFLICT OF INTEREST

The author confirms that this chapter has no conflict of interest.

ACKNOWLEDGEMENTS

None declared.

REFERENCES

[1] Udwadia ZF, Amale RA, Ajbani KK, Rodrigues C. Totally drug-resistant tuberculosis in India. Clin Infect Dis 2012; 54(4): 579-81.
[http://dx.doi.org/10.1093/cid/cir889] [PMID: 22190562]

[2] Farga V, Caminero JA. Tuberculosis. (3rd Ed.), Santiago de Chile: Editorial Mediterráneo 2011.

[3] Kant S, Maurya AK, Kushwaha RA, Nag VL, Prasad R. Multi-drug resistant tuberculosis: an iatrogenic problem. Biosci Trends 2010; 4(2): 48-55.
[PMID: 20448341]

[4] Curry International Tuberculosis Center and California Department of Public Health. Drug-Resistant Tuberculosis: A Survival Guide for Clinicians. (2nd ed.), 2011.

[5] Müller B, Borrell S, Rose G, Gagneux S. The heterogeneous evolution of multidrug-resistant *Mycobacterium tuberculosis*. Trends Genet 2013; 29(3): 160-9.
[http://dx.doi.org/10.1016/j.tig.2012.11.005] [PMID: 23245857]

[6] Uplekar M, Lönnroth K. MDR and XDR - the price of delaying engagement with all care providers for control of TB and TB/HIV. Trop Med Int Health 2007; 12(4): 473-4.
[http://dx.doi.org/10.1111/j.1365-3156.2007.01839.x] [PMID: 17445137]

[7] Andrews JR, Shah NS, Gandhi N, Moll T, Friedland G. Tugela Ferry Care and Research (TF CARES) Collaboration. Multidrug-resistant and extensively drug-resistant tuberculosis: implications for the HIV epidemic and antiretroviral therapy rollout in South Africa. J Infect Dis 2007; 196 (Suppl. 3): S482-90.
[http://dx.doi.org/10.1086/521121] [PMID: 18181698]

CHAPTER 4

Clinical Diagnosis of Drug Resistant Tuberculosis

Abstract: This chapter deals with the clinical diagnosis of drug resistant tuberculosis. Clinical detection of drug resistant tuberculosis requires a high index of suspicion by the clinician based in the information obtained from clinical records and the patient's medical history. Underlying drug resistance must be considered in patients who have been previously treated for TB, especially if there is a history of inadequate treatment regimen, in patients who are not showing significant clinical improvement or lack of bacteriological conversion, in contacts of a known drug resistant case and in chronic cases with a history of multiple treatment regimens. Required information includes a detailed clinical history of past tuberculosis episodes, name, dose and time a particular drug was taken by the patient, adverse reactions while under treatment, previous image studies for comparison purposes and all previous bacteriological studies available from clinical or laboratory records. The initial evaluation must include a thorough physical examination and basic laboratory tests (hemogram, blood chemistry, viral panel for hepatitis and HIV), audiometry, new chest x-rays and obtaining appropriate samples for complete bacteriological studies.

Keywords: Audiometry, Bacteriological conversion, Blood chemistry, Chest x-rays, Clinical, Diagnosis, Hemogram, Hepatitis B, Hepatitis C, HIV, Medical history, Physical examination, Previous treatment.

INTRODUCTION

Clinical detection of drug resistant tuberculosis requires a high index of suspicion by the clinician, a suspicion based in the information obtained from clinical records (when available) and the medical history during the patient clinical evaluation. It is of the utmost importance to identify through culture and drug susceptibility testing a drug resistant case as early as possible to start an effective drug regimen, to avoid the development of further resistance and to stop the transmission of a resistant strain in the community.

Rafael Laniado-Laborín

Clinical Classification of Drug Resistant Cases [1 - 4]

New Case:

Patient has never been treated with antituberculosis drugs (or has received them for less than a month)

Relapse:

Is defined as a patient who has become (and remained) culture negative while receiving therapy but after completion of therapy becomes culture positive again or has clinical or radiographic deterioration that is consistent with active tuberculosis.

Default:

Patients that interrupted treatment for one or more months

Failure:

Patient that while under treatment persist with positive culture by the end of the fourth month of treatment

Initial Case Evaluation

When evaluating a case with suspicion of drug resistance the following information must be obtained and documented:

- Demographic data (name, address/phone number when available, date of birth, country of birth, *etc.*)
- Detailed clinical history of past tuberculosis episodes: how many times the patient has been treated, where the patient was treated, name, dose and time (months or years) a particular drug was taken by the patient. This information is vital when deciding a new treatment regimen. Also it is important to obtain information about complications while under treatment (adverse reaction to antituberculosis treatment), surgical procedures, *etc.* If possible all this information should be confirmed from available medical records
- Chest radiograph: beside obtaining a new chest radiograph, every effort should be made to obtain previous studies for comparison purposes
- Other relevant information: co-morbidities and associated treatment drugs (diabetes,

hepatitis B or C, *etc.*), allergies, HIV status, illicit drug use, imprisonment, *etc.*

- Contact investigation (household, work, social)
- Thorough physical examination, including vital signs, weight and height
- Audiometry if injectable second drugs will be included in the regimen
- Basal blood exams: hemogram (CBC: red and white cell count, platelets), renal function (serum creatinine, creatinine depuration, BUN), liver function (ALT, AST, LDH, albumin), serum electrolytes, thyroid function tests (if prothionamide or PAS are included in the regimen)
- HIV testing
- Hepatitis B and C serology for subjects with history of intravenous drug use
- Pregnancy test for women in reproductive age

Underlying drug resistance must be considered if:

- patients who have been previously treated for TB, especially if there is a history of inadequate treatment regimen (defaulted, irregular drug intake, unsupervised treatment, *etc.*)
- patients who are not showing significant clinical improvement
- lack of bacteriological conversion (positive cultures after 4 months of treatment)
- immigrants from regions with high rates of drug resistant tuberculosis
- contacts of a known drug resistant case
- chronic cases with a history of multiple treatment regimens

Every effort should be made to obtain any existing clinical record of previous diagnosis and treatment. It is vital to determine if previous episodes where confirmed by mycobacterial culture and if drug susceptibility testing results are available.

Regarding previous treatment regimens we need to Know:

- When the patient was treated (when did treatment started and when it ended)?
- Where the patient was treated (it might be possible to obtain medical records)?
- What drugs where used (patient might not remember the names but might recall color and size of the pills, if they where injectables, *etc.*)?
- While under treatment did sputum became negative?
- How long did the patient received treatment?
- Was treatment strictly supervised?
- Was drug intake irregular with intermittencies?

- Did the patient finished the treatment regimen or defaulted?
- If the patient defaulted, what was the reason (adverse drug reactions? alcoholism? drug addiction?)
- How long after being discharged as cured did the symptoms reappear?

In patients with a history of more than one treatment, this information must be obtained for each previous treatment regimen. This information can be organized in a spreadsheet according to initial and final date each drug was taken.

CONFLICT OF INTEREST

The author confirms that this chapter has no conflict of interest.

ACKNOWLEDGEMENTS

None declared.

REFERENCES

[1] Curry International Tuberculosis Center and California Department of Public Health. Drug Resistant Tuberculosis: A Survival Guide for Clinicians. (2nd ed.), 2011.

[2] Farga V, Caminero JA. Tuberculosis. (3rd ed.), Santiago de Chile: Editorial Mediterraneo 2011.

[3] Guía para la Atención de Personas con Tuberculosis Resistente a Fármacos. Secretaria de Salud. Primera Edición 2010.

[4] Systematic screening for active tuberculosis: principles and recommendations. World Health Organization 2013. ISBN 9789241548601

CHAPTER 5

Drug Resistant Tuberculosis: Laboratory Diagnosis

Abstract: This chapter covers the available techniques for the diagnosis of tuberculosis (TB) and drug resistant tuberculosis. Definite diagnosis of tuberculosis requires the isolation on culture or the identification by molecular biology methods of *M. tuberculosis* (*Mtb*). Resistance to antituberculosis drugs, once *Mtb* has been identified can be carried through conventional culture methods (phenotypic methods) or molecular biology (genotypic methods). Ideally, susceptibility to at least isoniazid and rifampin should be carried in every case, especially in regions with high burden of drug resistant TB. The World Health Organization (WHO) recommends that at least 20% of all new cases and 100% of previously treated patients should be tested for drug resistance. Although the isolation of *Mtb* in cultures is still considered as the gold standard, advances in the field of molecular biology allows for a much rapid identification of *Mtb*, with excellent sensitivity and specificity. Drug susceptibility testing by phenotypic methods can be carried out in both solid and liquid media, but this process is slow, especially with the time-honored proportions method; we now have available molecular biology methods with excellent reliability for isoniazid and rifampin with results in a matter of hours.

Keywords: Antibiotics, Assay, Automated, BACTEC, Culture, DST, Drug-resistance, Isolation, Isoniazid, PCR, MGIT, MODS, Molecular, *M. tuberculosis*, Rifampin.

INTRODUCTION

Definite diagnosis of tuberculosis requires the isolation on culture or the identification by molecular biology methods of *M. tuberculosis (Mtb)*. Identification of *Mycobacterium tuberculosis* complex is vital as the first step in laboratory diagnosis. Nontuberculous mycobacteria (NTM) are genetically resistant to most antituberculosis drugs and since they are also acid-fast in microscopy a case could be mistakenly diagnosed as tuberculosis. There are several techniques for the identification of *Mtb*. Traditional biochemical testing

Rafael Laniado-Laborín

(niacin, catalase inhibition, and nitrate reduction) has a turnaround time of several weeks and has been displaced by several rapid tests: commercial genetic probes (Gen-Probe Amplified MTD, Gene-Probe®, San Diego, California), automated real time PCR (GeneXpert®, Cepheid, Sunnyvale, CA), a lateral chromatography rapid test for the MGIT system (MGIT TBc ID™ identification test, Becton Dickinson) among others.

Ideally, susceptibility to at least isoniazid and rifampin should be carried in every case, especially in regions with high burden of drug resistant TB. The World Health Organization (WHO) recommends that at least 20% of all new cases and 100% of previously treated patients should be tested for drug resistance. If resistance to rifampin (R) is proven the case is classified as pre-MDR (approximately 80% of R resistant cases are also resistant to isoniazid), and susceptibility tests for fluoroquinolones and second lines injectables should be requested to rule out as soon as possible the presence of an XDR-TB strain, and allow treatment with an efficient regimen avoiding the development of further resistance [1].

The traditional method of culture isolation of *Mtb* is still considered as the gold standard for diagnosis. The proportions method described by Canetti [2] allows for drug susceptibility testing (DST) for most of the first (FLD) and second line drugs (SLD), but it requires from 8 to 12 weeks, a major disadvantage for the treating clinician.

The BACTEC MGIT 960® system (Mycobacterial Growth Indicator Tube 960®, Becton Dickinson), is an automated method that has become a standard method for detection of drug resistance to FLD, (excluding pyrazinamide). It uses liquid media (Middlebrook 7 H9) with a fluorescent sensor to detect bacterial growth. Depending on the bacterial load in the sample cultivated, it takes an average of 3 weeks from time of inoculation to reporting of drug susceptibility [3]. Mycobacteria are first isolated in pure culture from clinical specimens (at this time identification with the MGIT TBc ID™ will take only 15 minutes), followed by inoculation of drug-containing broth (indirect method). It is possible to inoculate drug containing media directly with processed samples of AFB positive sputa (direct method); results of FLD DST will available in less than two weeks

[4]. However, the direct method for DST has a much higher rate of contaminated cultures resulting in failure rates up to 15% and therefore is rarely used. One important limitation of BACTEC MGIT 960® system is the high cost of the reagents. Because of its higher rate of contamination, cultures on liquid media should always have the backup of simultaneous cultures on solid media (*e.g.* Lowenstein-Jensen media and Stonebrink media in regions with high prevalence of disease by *Mycobacterium bovis*) [5].

Rapid Phenotypic DST Methods

There are some low cost phenotypic methods for DST that the WHO recently validated. These methods for rapid detection of resistance include the MODS assay and the nitrate reductase assay (NRA; Griess method).

The NRA (Griess method) is carried out in solid media supplemented with sodium or potassium nitrate as indicator of growth. Mtb possesses an **enzyme** (nitro-reductase) that reduces nitrate to nitrite; this reaction will produce a change in the color of the media (green in Lowenstein Jensen media) to red-purple when the Griess reagent is added to the media (Fig. **5.1**). The change in color in the media with an antibiotic means that the strain is resistant to this particular drug. Susceptibility to FLD can be determined in 8-10 days after obtaining a positive culture [6].

The Microscopic-Observation Drug-Susceptibility (MODS) assay uses liquid media (7H9 supplemented with OACD) in 24-well tissue-culture plates containing a combination of antibiotics (PANTA: polymixin, amphotericin B, nalidixic acid, trimethoprim and azlocillin) to prevent contamination with bacteria and fungi; antituberculosis drugs are added to media that then inoculated with the sputum sample; 12 wells are used: 4 control wells with no drugs, and two different concentrations of 4 antituberculosis drugs being tested in the remaining 8 wells. The cultures are examined under an inverted light microscope. Positive cultures are identified by cord formation, characteristic of *M. tuberculosis* growth in liquid media. The average time to culture positivity (and DST results) is about a week. Unlike other rapid methods the results of MODS are not affected by smear status [7].

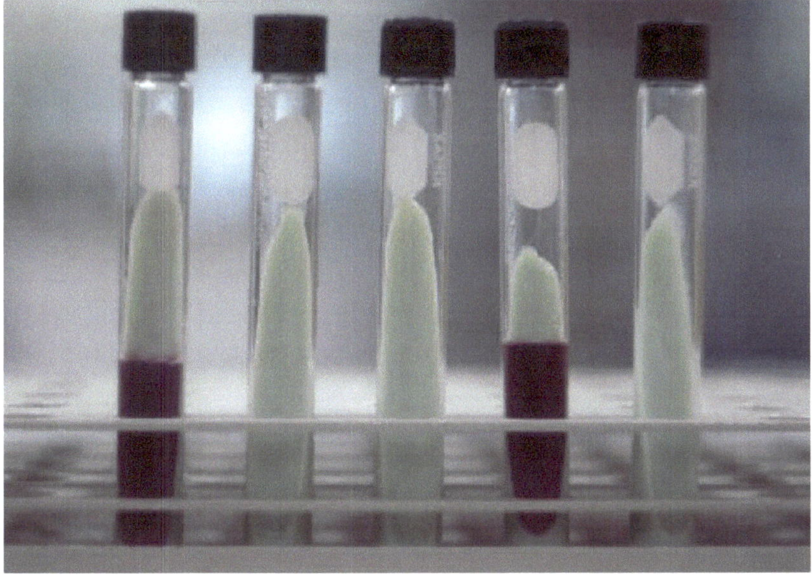

Fig. (5.1). Nitrate Reductase Assay (NRA or Griess method) showing a 670 strain resistant to rifampin (first tube from left is control, fourth is rifampin).

Although both the Griess and MODS are categorized as "rapid methods" and certainly are faster than the traditional proportions method, it still takes at least a couple of weeks for DST results. Nonetheless, taking into account their technical simplicity and low cost they are valuable tools for the diagnosis of DR-TB in developing countries.

Rapid Genotypic DST

Because *Mtb* drug resistance is genetically encoded, drug resistance by molecular methods can be detected in matter of hours. However, only a few resistance conferring mutations have been identified so far and phenotypic methods for DST are still required for most drugs.

The GenoTypeMTBDRPlus® (HAIN LIFESCIENCE, Nehren, Germany) can detect resistance to isoniazid (H) and rifampin (R) in sputum samples within 24 hours by detecting mutations in the katG and inhA genes for H and rpoB gene for R. The sensitivity and specificity for rifampin resistance is reported over 98%; sensitivity and specificity for H is lower due to the existence of other mutations that also confer resistance to H but cannot be detected by the assay. It is important to mention that there is a small proportion of mutations associated with resistance to R outside the *rpoB* gene that will not be detected with GenoTypeMTBDRPlus®; these mutations associated to both H and R will be detected through phenotypic methods [8]. There is an assay (GenoTypeMTBDRPlus®) designed to detect mutations in the genes gyrA, rrs and embB, mutations associated to resistance to fluoroquinolones, second line injectables (amikacin/capreeomicyn) and ethambutol respectively. However, the sensitivity has proven to be unacceptably low and the WHO does not recommend its use. The limitations of the GenoTypeMTBDRPlus® are the need of a molecular biology laboratory, trained personnel and the high cost of the reagents.

The GeneXpertMTB/RIF® (GeneXpert system, Cepheid, Sunnyvale, California) is an automated molecular test for *Mtb* species identification and rifampin resistance. Sensitivity of the GeneXpertMTB/RIF® assay is >98% for smear positive and >70% for smear negative cases; its specificity is >99% in patients without TB (Fig. **5.2**). Obviously, the positive and negative predictive values of this assay will vary depending on the regional prevalence of tuberculosis.

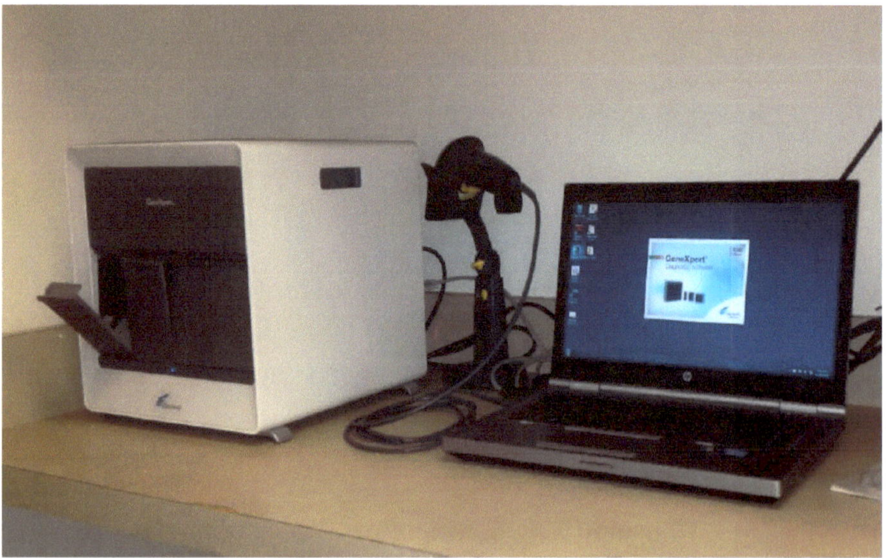

Fig. (5.2). A four cartridge XpertMTB/RIF® system connected to a laptop 723 computer (Cepheid, Sunnyvale, California).

This assay is designed for use at patient point of care and requires minimal personnel training. It needs only one manual step (sputum liquefaction/in-activation with a reagent and its transfer into the test cartridge); the disposable cartridge integrates real-time PCR technology that will allow the identification of *Mtb* and detection of mutations in the rpoB gen. The analysis is completed automatically by the instrument in about 2 hours.

The method was endorsed by WHO 2010 and a policy statement was released in 2011 [9]. Although initially the price of the equipment and cartridges were high and precluded its use in developing countries, prices were negotiated between international donors, a nonprofit organization and the producer, reducing the cost per test for public institutions from a list of 145 countries with high burden of MDR-TB and low income economies. The XpertMTB/Rif allows for immediate and highly accurate diagnosis of TB and detection of resistance to R in regions with high rates of TB and drug resistant TB; as mentioned, resistance to rifampin is a strong predictor of MDR-TB. A limitation of the Xpert is that it only detects resistance to rifampin and that like the GenoTypeMTBDRplus it will not detect mutations that occur outside of the rpoB core region [10].

An important issue that must be taking into account when interpreting DST results is the reproducibility of the assays depending on what drug is being tested (Table **5.1**). Results *in vitro* do not always coincide with the effectiveness *in vivo* of a given drug. Basically, DSTA's for isoniazid and rifampin are sensitive, specific and reproducible. DST for streptomycin and ethambutol are less reliable. Results for pyrazinamide are even more variable, especially with the automated methods. For second line drugs (SLD), DST for fluoroquinolones (levofloxacin and moxifloxacin) and injectables (kanamycin, amikacin and capreomycin) are the most reproducible. Reproducibility of phenotypic drug testing for other SLD (ethionamide, prothionamide, cycloserine, terizidone, p-aminosalicylic acid, clofazimine, amoxicillin/clavulanate, clari-thromycin, and linezolid) is poor and varies from one laboratory to another [11]. In general only national and supranational laboratories have the infrastructure and expertise to carry out second line drugs DST.

Table 5.1. Sensitivity and specificity of drug susceptibility assays for isoniazid and rifampin.

	Sensitivity isoniazid (%)	Specificity isoniazid (%)	Sensitivity rifampin (%)	Specificity rifampin (%)
NRA	94	100	99	100
MODS	92	96	96	96
GenoType plus	96	100	98	99

In conclusion, we now have several options for rapid diagnosis of DR-TB that complement the traditional phenotypic methods. Due to the rapid evolution of molecular biology we can expect new assays with higher sensitivity and specificity at affordable prices in the near future. Countries with high burden of drug resistant tuberculosis will have to evaluate the cost-benefit of implementing these new techniques to significantly reduce the time to diagnosis compared with traditional methods; this will allow the clinicians to select the most appropriate treatment regimen for a drug resistant case preventing the extension of resistance and its associated morbidity and mortality as well as limit the transmission of resistant strains in the community, a fundamental factor towards the overall control of drug resistant tuberculosis.

CONFLICT OF INTEREST

The author confirms that this chapter has no conflict of interest.

ACKNOWLEDGEMENTS

None declared.

REFERENCES

[1] Laniado-Laborin R, Palmero DJ, Caminero-Luna JA. Diagnosis and Treatment of Multidrug-Resistant Tuberculosis in Develop and Developing Countries: Finally Towards Equality. Curr Respir Med Rev 2012; 8: 464-74.
[http://dx.doi.org/10.2174/157339812804871292]

[2] Canetti G, Rist N, Grosset J. [Measurement of sensitivity of the tuberculous bacillus to antibacillary drugs by the method of proportions. Methodology, resistance criteria, results and interpretation]. Rev Tuberc Pneumol (Paris) 1963; 27: 217-72.
[PMID: 14018284]

[3] Siddiqi SH, Libonati JP, Middlebrook G. Evaluation of rapid radiometric method for drug

susceptibility testing of *Mycobacterium tuberculosis*. J Clin Microbiol 1981; 13(5): 908-12. [PMID: 6787076]

[4] Siddiqi S, Ahmed A, Asif S, *et al.* Direct drug susceptibility testing of *Mycobacterium tuberculosis* for rapid detection of multidrug resistance using the Bactec MGIT 960 system: a multicenter study. J Clin Microbiol 2012; 50(2): 435-40. [http://dx.doi.org/10.1128/JCM.05188-11] [PMID: 22162558]

[5] Laniado-LaborA-n R, MuA iz-Salazar R, GarcA-a-Ortiz RA, Vargas-Ojeda AC, Villa-Rosas C, Oceguera-Palao L. Molecular characterization of *Mycobacterium bovis* isolates from patients with tuberculosis in Baja California, Mexico. Infect Genet Evol 2014; 27: 1-5. [http://dx.doi.org/10.1016/j.meegid.2014.06.020] [PMID: 24997332]

[6] Solis LA, Shin SS, Han LL, Llanos F, Stowell M, Sloutsky A. Validation of a rapid method for detection of *M. tuberculosis* resistance to isoniazid and rifampin in Lima, Peru. Int J Tuberc Lung Dis 2005; 9(7): 760-4. [PMID: 16013771]

[7] Moore DA, Evans CA, Gilman RH, *et al.* Microscopic-observation drug-susceptibility assay for the diagnosis of TB. N Engl J Med 2006; 355(15): 1539-50. [http://dx.doi.org/10.1056/NEJMoa055524] [PMID: 17035648]

[8] Palomino JC. Current developments and future perspectives for TB diagnostics. Future Microbiol 2012; 7(1): 59-71. [http://dx.doi.org/10.2217/fmb.11.133] [PMID: 22191447]

[9] WHO. Policy statement: automated real-time nucleic acid amplification technology for rapid and simultaneous detection of tuberculosis and rifampin resistance: Xpert MTB/RIF system WHO/HTM/TB/2011.4.

[10] Boehme CC, Nabeta P, Hillemann D, *et al.* Rapid molecular detection of tuberculosis and rifampin resistance. N Engl J Med 2010; 363(11): 1005-15. [http://dx.doi.org/10.1056/NEJMoa0907847] [PMID: 20825313]

[11] World Health Organization (WHO). Policy Framework for Implementing New Tuberculosis Diagnostics 2010.

CHAPTER 6

Antituberculosis Drugs

Abstract: This chapter includes a comprehensive review of all drugs to treat tuberculosis. The WHO has classified these drugs in five groups, with drugs in Group 1 being the most effective, and less toxic and drugs in Group 5 being drugs with unproven efficacy or frequent side effects and/or toxicity. Each drug is discussed in detail, including its mechanisms of action, suggested doses and side and adverse effects, as well as the required clinical and laboratory monitoring for each drug. Recently added drugs bedaquiine and delamanid are also included in this review.

Keywords: Adverse effects, Antituberculosis drugs, Bedaquiline, Cycloserine, Delamanid, Dose, Effectiveness, Ethambutol, Ethionamide, Fluroquinolones, Injectables, Isoniazid, Laboratory, Linezolid, Monitoring, PAS, Pyrazinamide, Rifampin, Toxicity, WHO .

INTRODUCTION

The WHO has classified the antituberculosis drugs in five groups [1 - 3], with drugs in Group 1 being the most effective, and less toxic and drugs in Group 5 being drugs with unproven efficacy or frequent side effects and/or toxicity [4].

GROUP 1 DRUGS: FIRST LINE ORAL ANTITUBERCULOSIS DRUGS

Isoniazid (H)

Isoniazid is a potent bactericidal drug against *M. tuberculosis*, especially during the first few days of treatment exercising its maximal effect on mycobacteria with high metabolic rates. It blocks the synthesis of mycolic acid, a vital component of the mycobacterial wall leading to cell death. It is extremely effective against the large population of extracellular and intracavitary mycobacteria, rapidly reducing infectiousness.

It is recommended at a dose of 5 mg/kg/day orally (PO) up to a maximum of 300

Rafael Laniado-Laborín

mg/day. In children H is recommended at a dose of 10-15 mg/kg up to 300 mg daily (or 20-30 mg/kg two or three times a week). High dose H (16-18 mg/kg) has been used in patients with low-level resistance to H in the DST.

H is inactivated in the liver through acetylation and it can exacerbate liver damage if already present and cause hepatitis in patients without pre-existing liver disease. Liver enzymes (alanine transaminase [ALT] and aspartate transaminase [AST]) will increase in 10-20% of patients without clinical significance (<3 times the upper limit of normal) and does not require stopping the treatment.

H does not need dose adjustment in patients with renal failure.

H has a pharmacological interaction with phenytoin and carbamazepine increasing serum levels of both drugs.

Vitamin B6 (50-100 mg PO daily) should be added to the drug regimen in patients with risk of polyneuritis (diabetes, malnutrition, alcoholism, pregnancy) and in patients receiving high doses of H.

Absorption is better with an empty stomach; food with high fat content decreases its absorption in up to 50%.

H is safe during pregnancy and breastfeeding.

Some strains of *M. tuberculosis* display low grade resistance to H (0.2 I1/4g/mL) but are susceptible at higher concentrations (1.0 I1/4g/mL). H can be used in these circumstances at high doses (900 mg three times a week). It should not be used in patients with strains displaying high degree of resistance who have failed in the past with an H containing regimen [5].

Adverse Effects:

1. Hepatitis (directly related to patient's age with increased frequency in older patients). It usually subsides after stopping the drug, but in some cases can lead to acute liver failure
2. Peripheral polyneuritis (prevented with vitamin B6)
3. Optic neuritis (infrequent)
4. Arthralgia (infrequent)

5. Drug induced lupus-like syndrome (infrequent)
6. Psychosis (infrequent)

Monitoring:

In patients receiving other hepatotoxic drugs (or in those with preexisting liver damage, *e.g.* chronic viral hepatitis) liver function tests should be obtained at the start of treatment and then periodically (monthly) thereafter. Serum levels of H are recommended only in patients with suspected malabsorption or those with delayed bacteriological conversion.

Ethambutol (E)

Ethambutol is a bacteriostatic drug (inhibits cell wall synthesis) for oral use. Its importance resides in the fact that when used in a multiple drug regimen it will delay the development of resistance. The recommended dose is 15-25 mg/kg/day. In patients with multidrug resistant TB it should be started with the higher dose. Its absorption is not affected by food. Since it is eliminated through the kidneys, a dose of 30 mg/kg three times a week and serum levels are recommended in patients with renal failure to reduce the probability of serious adverse effects. No dose adjustment is required in patients with liver failure.

Adverse Effects:

1. Optic neuritis (dose-dependent). It is its more frequent adverse effect characterized by a decrease is visual acuity and the ability to discriminate red and green colors. Drug must be stopped immediately because damage is usually irreversible
2. Hypersensitivity
3. Peripheral paresthesia
4. Nausea, vomiting, anorexia, abdominal pain
5. Headache, dizziness

Monitoring:

Visual acuity and color discrimination (Snellen and Ishihara tests; Fig. **6.1**) at start of treatment and monthly thereafter.

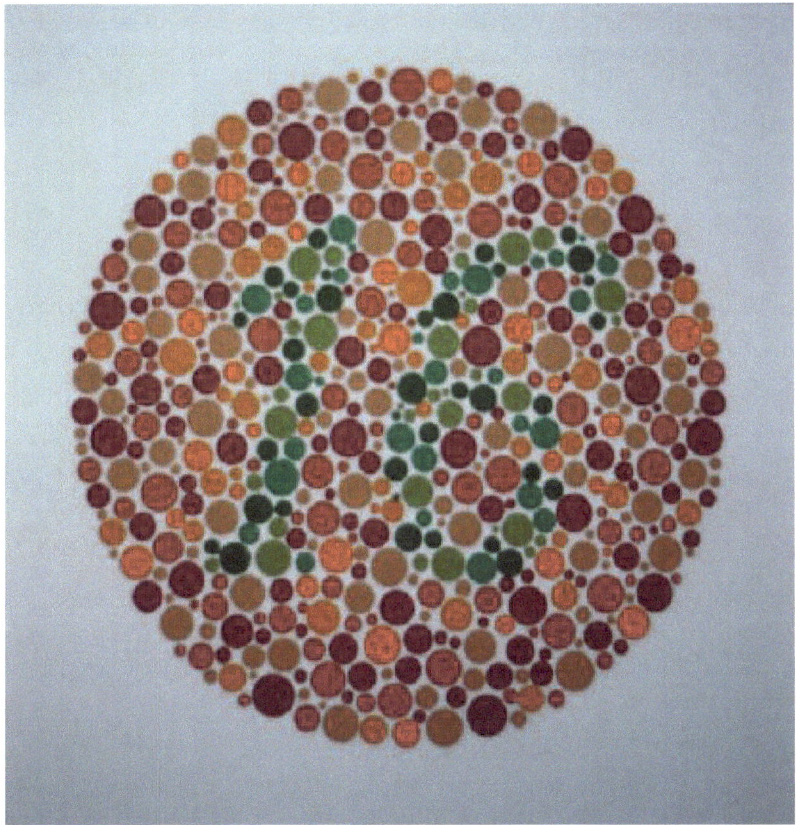

Fig. (6.1). Example of an Ishihara color test plate.

Pyrazinamide (Z)

It is a pro-drug, a synthetic derivate of nicotinamide (the amide of nicotinic acid, vitamin B3 or niacin) with bactericidal effect against *M. tuberculosis*, especially in an environment with acid pH, displaying sterilizing activity against intracellular bacilli.

The enzyme pyrazinamidase converts pyrazinamide to active pyrazinoic acid that accumulates inside the bacteria and inhibits fatty acids synthesis. Also, pyrazinoic acid binds to the ribosomal protein S1 and inhibits trans-translation explaining its ability to kill latent mycobacteria [6]. *Mycobacterium bovis* is genetically resistant to pyrazinamide.

The recommended dose of Z is 25 mg/kg/day PO (maximum daily dose is 2 grams); in children the daily dose is 20-40 mg/kg. Absorption is not affected by food. Z is eliminated through the kidney.

Adverse Effects:

1. Gout (infrequent) and arthralgia due to hyperuricemia; Z interferes with the renal excretion of uric acid.
2. Hepatotoxicity
3. Photosensitivity: patient should avoid exposure to sunlight and use sunscreen
4. Nausea, vomiting, anorexia
5. Hypersensitivity

Monitoring:

Monthly levels of uric acid.

Rifampin (R)

Synthetic drug from the rifamycin class, bactericidal against *M. tuberculosis* by inhibiting the synthesis of deoxyribonucleic acid (DNA). It is the most potent sterilizing drug available for TB, being very active against latent bacilli in necrotic lesions; it displays cross resistance with other rifamycins.

Recommended dose is 10 mg/kg/day up to a maximum of 600mg PO; it can be taken after meals but fatty food will decrease its absorption. In children the recommended dose is 10-20 mg/kg/day up to 600 mg/day. It is important to explain to the patient that urine, feces, tears, sweat, *etc.* will acquire a red/orange color. It does not require adjustment in patients with renal failure. It is inactivated in the liver and excreted through the bile pathway. R can cause hepatic damage and must be carefully monitored in patient with pre-existing liver disease.

R is a potent inductor of liver enzymes related to cytochrome P-450 and will increase the metabolism and half-life of several other drugs (oral diabetes drugs, anticoagulants, digitalis, contraceptives, *etc.*). This effect represent an important issue in patients with HIV co-infection who are receiving antiretroviral (ARV) treatment, especially those under treatment with protease inhibitors (*e.g.* ritonavir) and non-nucleoside reverse transcriptase inhibitors (NNRTIs like efavirenz or nevirapine), where rifampin will decrease the serum levels of the ARV drugs leading to ARV resistance. Since patients with MDR-TB are not going to receive rifampin the interaction of ARV drugs with the TB drug regimen does not represent a problem; however patients with mono or poly-resistance might be treated with rifampin and will need to modify their ARV regimen.

Rifampin is safe during pregnancy and breastfeeding. An alternative contraception method will be needed in patients of child-bearing age because rifampin will decrease the blood level of oral contraceptives.

Adverse Effects:

1. Hepatotoxicity (frequency will increase when administered with other hepatotoxic drugs like H and Z). It consists of cholestatic jaundice (without elevation of liver enzymes) or drug induced hepatitis with jaundice and elevated liver enzymes (AST and especially ALT) >3 times the serum normal upper limit
2. Hemolytic anemia, thrombocytopenia
3. Urticaria
4. Dyspepsia
5. *Flu-like syndrome*, (especially when administered in a non-daily regimen

Monitoring:

Monthly hemoglobin levels, liver function tests (in patients with liver damage). Serum drug levels might be necessary if the patient is receiving other drugs that affect rifampin liver metabolism (*e.g.* antiretroviral drugs).

GROUP 2 DRUGS [7, 8]

Second Line Injectables

Amikacin (Am)

Semi-synthetic aminoglycoside with bactericidal activity. It displays cross resistance with kanamycin and to a lesser degree with capreomycin. Recommended dose is 15 mg/kg/day (up to 1 gr. daily in adults) 5-7 times per week; in patients >60 years of age the recommended dose is 10 mg/kg/day (up to 750 mg/day). Once sputum culture becomes negative, it can be spaced to 3 times per week. It can be administered intramuscular (IM) or intravenous (IV). For IV administration it must be diluted in 100 mL of 5% dextrose solution.

Amikacin can produce fetal deafness and it should not be used during pregnancy. Can be used while breastfeeding. In patients with renal failure, interval adjustment (12-15 mg/ kg dose 2-3 times a week) is recommended and serum drug levels must be monitored periodically. There is no need for dose adjustment in patients with liver disease. Concomitant use of loop diuretic will increase the risk of ototoxicity.

Adverse Reactions:

1. Nephrotoxicity: directly related to dose and duration of regimen (higher doses and prolonged administration increase the risk of renal toxicity
2. Ototoxicity: increased with prolonged used; risk is higher in older subjects
3. Electrolyte abnormalities: hypokalemia/hypomagnesemia
4. Vestibular toxicity with equilibrium disorders

Monitoring:

Monthly monitoring of renal function (creatinine and creatinine clearance in subjects with basal renal impairment and in subjects over 60 years of age) and electrolytes (including calcium and magnesium) is recommended. Perform monthly audiology and vestibular exams. Drug serum levels are recommended in patients with pre-existing renal impairment.

Capreomycin (Cm)

Bactericidal cyclic polypeptide that inhibits protein synthesis. Recommended dose is 15 mg/kg/day (up to 1 gr. daily in adults) 5-7 times per week; in patients >60 years of age the recommended dose is 10 mg/kg/day (up to 750 mg/day). Once sputum culture becomes negative, it can be spaced to 3 times per week. It can be administered intramuscular (IM) or intravenous (IV). For IV administration it must be diluted in 100 mL of 5% dextrose solution.

Capreomycin can produce fetal deafness and it should not be used during pregnancy. Can be used while breastfeeding. In patients with renal failure, interval adjustment (12-15 mg/ kg dose 2-3 times a week) is recommended and serum drug levels must be monitored periodically. There is no need for dose adjustment in patients with liver disease. Concomitant use of loop diuretic will increase the risk of ototoxicity.

Adverse Effects:

1. Nephrotoxicity: up to 20-25% of patients, including proteinuria, decreased creatinine clearance and electrolyte abnormalities.
2. Ototoxicity: increased with prolonged used; risk is higher in older subjects
3. Vestibular toxicity with risk of ataxia
4. Electrolyte abnormalities: hypokalemia/hypomagnesemia

Monitoring:

Monthly monitoring of renal function (creatinine and creatinine clearance in subjects with basal renal impairment and in subjects over 60 years of age) and electrolytes (including calcium and magnesium) is recommended. Perform monthly audiology and vestibular exams. Drug serum levels are recommended in patients with pre-existing renal impairment.

Kanamycin (Km)

Parental aminoglycoside, bactericidal. Cross resistance with amikacin and to a lesser degree with capreomycin but not with streptomycin

Recommended dose is 15 mg/kg/day (up to 1 gr. daily in adults) 5-7 times per week; in patients >60 years of age the recommended dose is 10 mg/kg/day (up to 750 mg/day). Once sputum culture becomes negative, it can be spaced to 3 times per week. It can be administered intramuscular (IM) or intravenous (IV). For IV administration it must be diluted in 100 mL of 5% dextrose solution.

In patients with renal failure, interval adjustment (12-15 mg/ kg dose 2-3 times a week) is recommended and serum drug levels must be monitored periodically. There is no need for dose adjustment in patients with liver disease. Concomitant use of loop diuretic will increase the risk of ototoxicity. Kanamycin can produce fetal deafness and it should not be used during pregnancy. Can be used while breastfeeding.

Adverse Effects:

1. Nephrotoxicity: more nephrotoxic than streptomycin
2. Ototoxicity: increased with prolonged used; risk is higher in older subjects
3. Vestibular toxicity with risk of ataxia (slightly less than other injectables)
4. Electrolyte abnormalities: hypokalemia/hypomagnesemia

Monitoring:

Monthly monitoring of renal function (creatinine and creatinine clearance in subjects with basal renal impairment and in subjects over 60 years of age) and electrolytes (including calcium and magnesium) is recommended. Perform monthly audiology and vestibular exams. Drug serum levels are recommended in patients with pre-existing renal impairment.

GROUP 3 DRUGS: FLUOROQUINOLONES

Gatifloxacin (Gfx)

Third generation bactericidal fluoroquinolone (FQ), highly active against *M. tuberculosis*. It kills MTB by inhibiting DNA gyrase.

The recommended dose (once a day) is 400 mg/day IV or PO.

Oral absorption is excellent, but dairy products, antacids, sucralfate, didanosine or supplements that contain iron, magnesium, zinc and calcium, should be avoided at least for two hours before and after the dose of Gfx.

Recommended dose in patients with renal failure is 200 mg after dialysis or 400 mg three times per week after dialysis.

Rarely associated with elevated transaminases. Its use during pregnancy and breastfeeding should be avoided due to observation of arthropathy in animal models.

Adverse Effects:

1. Nausea, bloating, diarrhea
2. Headaches, dizziness, insomnia, tremor

3. Tendon rupture (rare), arthralgias (avoid strenuous exercise)
4. QT interval prolongation (becomes important when combined with other drugs with the same toxicity (*e.g.* delamanid, bedaquiline)
5. Photosensitivity: avoid excessive exposure to sunlight and use sun blockers
6. Hypo or hyperglycemia. Should be avoided in patients with diabetes

Monitoring:

Clinical; does not require specific laboratory tests monitoring.

Levofloxacin (Lfx)

Third generation bactericidal fluoroquinolone (FQ), highly active against *M. tuberculosis*. It may display cross resistance with other FQ, although is not infrequent that it may retain its efficacy even when the strain is resistant to other FQ's. It is more potent than ciprofloxacin and ofloxacin. It kills MTB by inhibiting DNA gyrase.

The recommended dose (once a day) is 500-750 mg/day (if weight is less than 45 kg the recommended dose is 500 mg/day). Dose can be increased to 1 gr/day in cases with complicated resistance patterns. It can be administered PO or IV.

Oral absorption is excellent, but dairy products, antacids, sucralfate, didanosine or supplements that contain iron, magnesium, zinc and calcium, should be avoided at least for two hours before and after the dose of Lfx. Recommended dose in patients with renal failure is 750 mg-1 gr. three times a week. No adjustment is needed in patient with liver disease. Its use during pregnancy and breastfeeding should be avoided due to observation of arthropathy in animal models.

Adverse Effects:

1. Nausea, bloating, diarrhea
2. Headaches, dizziness, insomnia, tremor
3. Tendon rupture (rare), arthralgias (avoid strenuous exercise)
4. QT interval prolongation (becomes important when combined with other drugs with the same toxicity (*e.g.* delamanid, bedaquiline)
5. Photosensitivity: avoid excessive exposure to sunlight and use sun blockers

Monitoring:

Clinical; does not require specific laboratory tests monitoring.

Moxifloxacin (Mfx)

Fourth generation bactericidal FQ, highly active against *M. tuberculosis*. It may display cross resistance with other FQ, although is not infrequent that it may retain its efficacy even when the strain is resistant *in vitro* to other FQA's. Like other FQ it inhibits DNA gyrase.

Recommended dose is 400 mg once a day PO or IV. Oral absorption is excellent but dairy products, antacids, sucralfate, didanosine or supplements that contain iron, magnesium, zinc and calcium, should be avoided at least for two hours before and after the dose of Mfx. Does not require dose adjustment in patients with renal failure. Very rarely is associated with hepatotoxicity. Its use during pregnancy and while breastfeeding should be avoided due to observation of arthropathy in animal models.

Adverse Effects:

1. Nausea, bloating, diarrhea
2. Headaches, dizziness, insomnia, tremor
3. Tendon rupture (rare), arthralgias (avoid strenuous exercise)
4. QT interval prolongation (becomes important when combined with other drugs with the same toxicity (*e.g.* delamanid, bedaquiline)
5. Photosensitivity: avoid excessive exposure to sunlight and use sun blockers

Monitoring:

Clinical; does not require specific laboratory tests monitoring.

GROUP 4 DRUGS: SECOND LINE ORAL ANTITUBERCULOSIS DRUGS

Cycloserine (Cs)

Analog of d-alanin with bacteriostatic effect (inhibits peptidoglycan synthesis of the bacterial cell wall).

Recommended dose is 10-15 mg/kg/day PO (in adults 250 mg twice a day). Absorption is decreased by food. All patients treated with this drug should receive a supplement of vitamin B6 (50 mg per each 250 mg cycloserine dose).

It is cleared by the kidneys and will require dose adjustment (either 250 mg daily or 500 mg three times per week) and serum levels monitoring (adjusted to maintain between 20 and 25 μg/mL; Table **6.2**). No adjustment is needed in patients with liver damage. If there are no other options it may be used during pregnancy. It can be used while breast feeding, but the child must receive B6 supplement).

Table 6.2. Serum blood levels of antituberculosis drugs.

Drug	Daily dose	Usual serum Cmax
Isoniazid	300 mg	3-6 μg/ml
Rifampin	600 mg	8-24 μg/ml
Pyrazinamide	25 mg/kg	20-50 μg/ml
Ethambutol	25 mg/kg	2-6 μg/ml
PAS	4 G BID	20-60 μg/ml (granules)
Cycloserine	250 mg BID	25 to 30 μg/ml
Clofazimine	100 mg	0.5-2 μg/ml
Ethionamide	250 mg BID	0.99–6.1 μg/ml
Levofloxacin	500 mg	1.81–0.6 μg/ml
Moxifloxacin	400 mg	0.72-5.72 μg/ml

Modified from Peloquin CA [19].

Adverse Effects:

1. Central nervous system toxicity (CNS): (especially if serum levels >35 μg/mL). It is contraindicated in patients with a history of seizures, psychosis or alcoholism. Adverse effects include lethargy, lack of concentration, seizures, depression, psychotic episodes, suicidal ideation
2. Peripheral neuropathy
3. Lichenoid dermatitis
4. Exfoliative dermatitis (Stevens-Johnson syndrome)

Monitoring:

Clinical monitoring of CNS toxicity.

Ethionamide (Eth)

Derivative of isonicotinic acid, weakly bactericidal against *M. tuberculosis*; it blocks the synthesis of mycolic acids affecting the cell wall integrity. When the strain presents a mutation in the *inhA* gene conferring low grade resistance to isoniazid, it will frequently be also resistant to ethionamide.

The recommended dose of Eth is 15-20 mg/kg/day PO (in adults 500-750 mg divided in 2-3 doses. Oral absorption is not affected by food (Table **6.1**). It should be started at a dose of 250 mg/day and ramped up to 500 mg within a week to avoid adverse gastrointestinal effects. All patients must receive vitamin B6 (50 mg per every 250 mg of Eth), especially if the regimen also includes cycloserine.

Table 6.1. Effect of food on absorption of antituberculosis drugs and type of monitoring required.

DRUG	EFFECT OF FOOD ON ABSORPTION	MONITORING
Amikacin	Not affected	Renal function; audiometry and vestibular testing. Electrolytes
Amoxicillin/clavulanate	Not affected	No specific monitoring
Capreomycin	Not affected	Renal function; audiometry and vestibular testing. Electrolytes
Cycloserine	Decrease absorption Better absorption if fasting	Clinical monitoring of psychiatric symptoms
Clofazimine	Increased absorption with food	Clinical monitoring
Ethambutol	Not affected	Snellen and Ishihara testing
Ethionamide/Prothionamide	Not affected	Liver and thyroid function tests
Gatifloxacin	Avoid ingestion within 2 hours before and after the drug dose of dairy products (milk, cream, yogurt, *etc.*), dairy products, antacids, sucralfate, iron, magnesium, zinc, calcium, polyvitamins)	Clinical monitoring
Imipenem/cilastatin	Not affected	Clinical monitoring
Isoniazid	Decrease absorption with fatty foods	Liver function tests

(Table 6.1) contd.....

DRUG	EFFECT OF FOOD ON ABSORPTION	MONITORING
Kanamycin	Not affected	Renal function; audiometry and vestibular testing. Electrolytes
Levofloxacin	Avoid ingestion within 2 hours before and after the drug dose of dairy products (milk, cream, yogurt, *etc.*), dairy products, antacids, sucralfate, iron, magnesium, zinc, calcium, polyvitamins)	Clinical monitoring
Linezolid	Not affected	Clinical monitoring, Snellen and Ishihara testing, hemogram
Moxifloxacin	Avoid ingestion within 2 hours before and after the drug dose of dairy products (milk, cream, yogurt, *etc.*), dairy products, antacids, sucralfate, iron, magnesium, zinc, calcium, polyvitamins)	Clinical monitoring
PAS	Mix with applesauce or yogurt	Thyroid function tests, electrolytes, hemogram, liver function tests
Pyrazinamide	Not affected	Uric acid levels; liver function tests
Rifampin	Decrease absorption with fatty foods	Hemogram and liver function tests

Like H it can induce liver damage and it should be monitored closely in patients with preexisting liver damage. There is no need for dose adjustment in patients with renal failure. It should not be used during pregnancy because of its teratogenic potential; up to 20% of the dose will be excreted through maternal milk.

Adverse Effects:

1. Dyspepsia, anorexia, nausea, vomiting, sialorrhea and dysgeusia (metallic taste). This side effect can become intolerable; taking the dose after meals might lessen the symptoms
2. Hepatotoxicity
3. Gynecomastia, alopecia, acne, impotence, menstrual irregularity, hypothyroidism (reversible) that should be treated with replacement hormone
4. Neurotoxicity: depression, confusion, paresthesia
5. Hypersensitivity

Monitoring:

Bimonthly levels of thyroid stimulant hormone (TSH) to determine if hormone replacement is needed. Monthly liver function tests.

Para-Aminosalicylate (PAS)

Bacteriostatic agent with activity against *M. tuberculosis* by interfering with its folic acid synthesis.

Recommended dose is from 8 to twelve grams daily PO divided in 2-3 doses (children 200-300 mg/kg/day). It should be kept in the refrigerator. The granules can be mixed in applesauce or yogurt or with an acid beverage (orange, tomato, apple or grapefruit juice).

It does not require adjustment in patients with renal failure (an inactive metabolite is excreted in urine). There is no information regarding its safety during pregnancy or breastfeeding. Liver damage has been reported occasionally and it should be monitored closely in patients with pre-existing liver damage.

Adverse Effects:

1. Digestive especially diarrhea, nausea, vomiting, gastrointestinal bleeding
2. Hepatotoxicity (uncommon)
3. Coagulopathy (uncommon)
4. Reversible hypothyroidism (more frequent if administered on a regimen containing ethionamide/prothionamide)

Monitoring:

Monthly safety exams (electrolytes, hemogram, liver function tests). Thyroid function tests every two months.

GROUP 5 DRUGS: (WITH THE EXCEPTION OF LINEZOLID WITH VIRTUALLY NO EVIDENCE OF THEIR EFFICACY) [9]

Amoxicillin/Clavulanate (Amx/Clv)

Combination of penicillin and an inhibitor of β-lactamase for oral administration.

There is little evidence of its efficacy, but it could have early bactericidal activity. Recommended dose is 1 gram of amoxicillin and 250 mg of clavulanate three times a day. Absorption is not affected by food. Since amoxicillin is cleared through the kidneys, in patients with renal failure and creatinine clearance <30 mL/min dose must be reduced to 1 gr of amoxicillin once a day. Clavulanate is cleared through the liver so it must be used carefully in patients with liver damage.

Adverse Effects:

1. Diarrhea and abdominal pain
2. Nausea and vomiting
3. Cutaneous rash
4. Hypersensitivity (should be used with precaution in patients referring allergy to β-lactamic antibiotics

Monitoring:

Does not require specific monitoring.

Clofazimine (Cfz)

Fat-soluble riminophenazine utilized in the treatment of leprosy and active *in vitro* against *M. tuberculosis*; however there is very little evidence of its clinical efficacy. The largest clinical study has been the Bangladesh trial, which included 427 subjects treated with a regimen that included Cfz, reporting a success rate of 75.6% [5]. It has been reserved for drug-resistant cases with no other options. Cfz works through effects on intracellular redox cycling and cell wall destabilization [10].

The recommended dose in adults is of 100 to 200 mg daily (oral). A regimen of 200 mg daily for 2 months, followed by 100 mg daily has been also suggested. In children, recommended dose is 1 mg/kg/day. Absorption is enhanced by food; highest bioavailability occurs when taken with fatty meals.

No dose change is needed in renal disease, but dose adjustment may be necessary in patients with severe hepatic impairment. There is no information on its safety during pregnancy; should be avoided while breastfeeding due to skin pigmentation of the infant.

Adverse Effects:

1. Gastrointestinal intolerance (nausea, vomiting, abdominal pain) in 50% of cases
2. Orange to brownish skin, conjunctival and corneal pigmentation (75-100%) of patients within a few weeks, as well as similar discoloration of most bodily fluids and secretions. This effect is reversible but may take months to years to disappear
3. Icthyosis and skin dryness (8–28%)
4. Photosensitivity (avoid sunlight and use sunscreen)

Monitoring:

No specific laboratory monitoring is recommended in patients receiving Cfz.

Imipenem/Cilastatin (Imp/Cln)

β-lactamic antibiotic (carbapenem class) for IV or IM administration. It has *in vitro* activity against *M. tuberculosis*, but there is very little clinical experience.

The combination of amoxicillin/clavulanate plus meropenem is active against MDR/XDR-TB *in vitro*, and this triple therapy could be a useful therapy for MDR/XDR-TB [11].

Recommended dose in adults is 1 g. twice a day. Meropenem at a dose of 20-40 mg/kg IV three times per day is preferred in children because there are reports of seizures with imipenem. The IM route is usually impractical due to the high dose and frequency required with these drugs.

Dose adjustment is required in patients with renal failure (creatinine clearance <30 mL/min). The recommended dose is 500 mg IV three times per day, or 500 mg twice a day in those with creatinine clearance <20 mL/min.

It should be use with caution in patients with a history of allergy to penicillin or cephalosporin and in those being treated with ganciclovir.

Adverse Effects:

1. Diarrhea, nausea, vomiting
2. Seizures (especially in patients with meningitis)
3. Hypersensitivity

Monitoring:

Symptomatic.

Meropenem (MER)

Meropenem is a β-lactamic antibiotic (carbapenem class) for IV administration. When combined with a β-lactamic inhibitor (*e.g.* clavulanate) it has *in vitro* bactericidal activity against *M. tuberculosis*, and in case series has shown promise in the treatment of patients with XDR-TB [12, 13]. Since it will be used for prolonged periods a central line is needed for its administration.

Recommended dose is 1 g. BID. Meropenem would be the drug of choice in children (at a dose of 20-40 mg/kg IV three times per day) because there are reports of seizures with imipenem.

Dose adjustment is required in patients with renal failure (creatinine clearance < 30 ml/min).

It should be use with caution in patients with a history of allergy to penicillin or cephalosporin and in those being treated with ganciclovir.

Adverse Effects:

1. Diarrhea, nausea, vomiting
2. Seizures (it can reduce the plasma concentration of valproic acid)
3. Hypersensitivity

Monitoring:

Symptomatic.

Linezolid (Lzd)

Oxazolidinone antibiotic with *in vitro* bactericidal effect against *M. tuberculosis* for oral or IV administration. Lzd inhibits protein synthesis of mycobacteria. It is considered the most effective of the group 5 drugs [14].

Recommended dose is 600 mg/day PO and absorption is not affected by food. In children the recommended dose is of 10 mg/kg three times per day. All patients must receive B6 supplement.

There are reports that linezolid blood levels increase after the co-administration of 500 mg of clarithromycin PO, compared to baseline. Co-administration is well tolerated by most patients [15].

Lzd does not require dose adjustment in patients with renal failure; liver damage is uncommon. There is no information regarding its safety during pregnancy or breastfeeding.

Patient should avoid foods and beverages containing tyramine (aged cheeses, dried meats, sauerkraut, soy sauce, tap beers, red wine) because it can trigger an hypertensive crisis.

Adverse Effects:

1. Myelosuppresion (anemia, leucopenia, thrombocytopenia)
2. Diarrhea, nausea, vomiting
3. Optic and peripheral neuropathy (uncommon)

Monitoring:

Hemogram (CBC) frequently during the initial period, followed by monthly exams. Monthly Snellen and Ishihara testing.

NEW DRUGS AVAILABLE FOR CLINICAL USE

Bedaquiline (BQ)

In December 2012, the FDA approved bedaquiline for its use in the United States as part of a multiple drug regimen (at least 4 active drugs) administered as DOT in adults ≥18 years diagnosed with multidrug resistant TB when there are no other drug options [7]. Usually drugs are approved by the FDA after testing in thousands of subjects; the total number of subjects included in bedaquiline clinical trials before its approval by the FDA was only 208 [16].

Bedaquiline is a diarylquinoline antituberculosis drug that blocks the proton pump of ATP synthetase of MTB, critical enzyme for synthesis of mycobacterial ATP. So far there is no cross resistance with any of the first line drugs, amikacin or moxifloxacin.

Bedaquiline is metabolized through the cytochrome P450 (CYP) system. Simultaneous administration of bedaquiline with rifamycins or other strong CYP3A4 inducers should be avoided if possible. There is no interaction with the antiretroviral nevirapine, but lopinavir/ritonavir (Kaletra™) increase bedaquiline plasma concentration up to 20%. No significant pharmacokinetic interactions have been reported between bedaquiline and isoniazid, pyrazinamide, ethambutol, kanamycin, or cycloserine.

Among the limited studies to date, no significant pharmacokinetic interactions have been observed between bedaquiline and the anti-TB drugs isoniazid, pyrazinamide, ethambutol, kanamycin, ofloxacin, or cycloserine.

Recommended dose is 400 mg PO once a day (100 mg tablets) for two weeks, followed by 200 mg PO three times per week for 24 weeks. Bioavailability is doubled when administered with fat rich food. Black subjects' clear bedaquiline 50% more rapidly than subjects from other races, with the consequent decrease plasma exposure.

Beaquiline has an extremely prolonged half-life (4-5 months) resistance could theoretically be acquired if the rest of the regimen is stopped too early and bedaquiline practically becomes monotherapy. For these reason the rest of the drugs in the regimen must be continued for at least 5 months after stopping bedaquiline.

There are no human studies in pregnant females, and animal studies show that it concentrates in maternal milk.

The main goal in the bedaquiline clinical trials was sputum culture conversion. Overall patients treated with bedaquiline converted cultures more rapidly than controls (78% *vs*. 58% at 24 weeks, p=0.014) but at the end of the trials there was significant difference among the groups (70% *vs*. 56%, p=0.09 at 72 weeks).

There was a 5-fold mortality rate in the BQ compared with placebo and 50% were due to tuberculosis; in some cases cause of death was not determined.

Adverse Effects:

1. Nausea, vomiting
2. Arthralgia
3. Headaches
4. Hyperuricemia
5. Liver damage
6. Q-T interval prolongation

a. QTc between 450-480 milliseconds: 26.6% for BQ *vs*. 8.6% for controls
b. increment of >60 ms: 9.1% for BQ *vs*. 2.5% for controls

Factors that increase the risk of prolonged Q-T interval

a. concomitant use of other drugs that prolong the Q-T interval (fluoroquinolones, macrolides, clofazimine)
b. History of torsade de pointes
c. Congenital prolonged Q-T syndromes
d. Hypothyroidism
e. Bradyarrhythmia
f. Low levels of calcium, magnesium or potassium

The FDA approved bedaquiline with a "black box" warning due to a higher mortality rate and the Q-T interval prolongation in patients treated with this drug in comparison with placebo.

Monitoring:

a. Clinical monitoring of adverse effects (nausea, headaches, arthralgia)
b. Monthly sputum culture
c. Monthly liver function tests

d. Electrocardiogram: basal and at 2, 12 and 24 weeks of treatment

Delamanid

Bactericidal derivate of nitrodihydro-imidazooxazole. Inhibits mycolic acid synthesis. Potent *in vitro* activity against drug-susceptible and drug resistant strains of MTB [17, 18]. It was approved by EMEA in November 2013.

In a multinational randomized double-blind, placebo-controlled trial, patients who received a background drug regimen plus 100 mg of delamanid twice daily, 45.4% achieved sputum culture conversion at 2 months, as compared with 29.6% of patients who received a background drug regimen plus placebo (p=0.008); as compared with the placebo group, the group that received the background drug regimen plus 200 mg of delamanid twice daily had a higher proportion of patients with sputum-culture conversion (41.9%, p=0.04) [9].

Adverse Effects:

1. Anemia
2. Nausea, vomiting, upper abdominal pain
3. Prolonged QT interval on electrocardiogram

Monitoring:

a. Electrocardiogram: basal and at 2, 12 y 24 weeks of treatment.
b. Monthly sputum culture.

CONCLUSIONS ON NEW DRUGS FOR MDR-TB

MDR and XDR patients treated with bedaquiline or delamanid (plus the WHO background regimen) show added benefit from the use of these drugs. However they share a troublesome and potentially lethal side effect (prolonged QT interval) among themselves and with other drugs used in the treatment of resistant tuberculosis (fluoroquinolones) and its simultaneous use is not recommended. Another important disadvantage is that both drugs are extremely expensive and most national TB programs will not be able to include them in treatment regimens (as has been the case with linezolid) of patients with disease due to *M. tuberculosis* strains with complex resistance patterns.

CONFLICT OF INTEREST

The author confirms that this chapter has no conflict of interest.

ACKNOWLEDGEMENTS

None declared.

REFERENCES

[1] Curry International Tuberculosis Center and California Department of Public Health. Drug-Resistant Tuberculosis: A Survival Guide for Clinicians. (2nd ed.), 2011.

[2] Farga V, Caminero JA. Tuberculosis. (3rd Ed.), Santiago de Chile: Editorial Mediterraneo 2011.

[3] Guía para la Atención de Personas con Tuberculosis Resistente a Fármacos. Secretaria de Salud. Primera Edición 2010.

[4] Guidelines for the programmatic management of drug-resistant tuberculosis – 2011 update. World Health Organization 2011. ISBN 978 92 4 150158 3.

[5] Katiyar SK, Bihari S, Prakash S, Mamtani M, Kulkarni H. A randomised controlled trial of high-dose isoniazid adjuvant therapy for multidrug-resistant tuberculosis. Int J Tuberc Lung Dis 2008; 12(2): 139-45.
[PMID: 18230245]

[6] Moulding T. A randomised controlled trial of high-dose isoniazid adjuvant therapy for multidrug-resistant tuberculosis. Int J Tuberc Lung Dis 2008; 12(9): 1102. [Letter].
[PMID: 18713512]

[7] Caminero JA, Sotgiu G, Zumla A, Migliori GB. Best drug treatment for multidrug-resistant and extensively drug-resistant tuberculosis. Lancet Infect Dis 2010; 10(9): 621-9.
[http://dx.doi.org/10.1016/S1473-3099(10)70139-0] [PMID: 20797644]

[8] Van Deun A, Maug AK, Salim MA, *et al.* Short, highly effective, and inexpensive standardized treatment of multidrug-resistant tuberculosis. Am J Respir Crit Care Med 2010; 182(5): 684-92.
[http://dx.doi.org/10.1164/rccm.201001-0077OC] [PMID: 20442432]

[9] Chang KC, Yew WW, Tam CM, Leung CC. WHO group 5 drugs and difficult multidrug-resistant tuberculosis: a systematic review with cohort analysis and meta-analysis. Antimicrob Agents Chemother 2013; 57(9): 4097-104.
[http://dx.doi.org/10.1128/AAC.00120-13] [PMID: 23774431]

[10] Gopal M, Padayatchi N, Metcalfe JZ, O'Donnell MR. Systematic review of clofazimine for the treatment of drug-resistant tuberculosis. Int J Tuberc Lung Dis 2013; 17(8): 1001-7.
[http://dx.doi.org/10.5588/ijtld.12.0144] [PMID: 23541151]

[11] Gonzalo X, Drobniewski F. Is there a place for I -lactams in the treatment of multidrug-resistant/extensively drug-resistant tuberculosis? Synergy between meropenem and amoxicillin/clavulanate. J Antimicrob Chemother 2013; 68(2): 366-9.
[http://dx.doi.org/10.1093/jac/dks395] [PMID: 23070734]

[12] De Lorenzo S, Alffenaar JW, Sotgiu G, *et al.* Efficacy and safety of meropenem-clavulanate added to linezolid-containing regimens in the treatment of MDR-/XDR-TB. Eur Respir J 2013; 41(6): 1386-92. [http://dx.doi.org/10.1183/09031936.00124312] [PMID: 22997218]

[13] Payen MC, De Wit S, Martin C, *et al.* Clinical use of the meropenem-clavulanate combination for extensively drug-resistant tuberculosis. Int J Tuberc Lung Dis 2012; 16(4): 558-60. [http://dx.doi.org/10.5588/ijtld.11.0414] [PMID: 22325421]

[14] Sotgiu G, Centis R, D'Ambrosio L, *et al.* Efficacy, safety and tolerability of linezolid containing regimens in treating MDR-TB and XDR-TB: systematic review and meta-analysis. Eur Respir J 2012; 40(6): 1430-42. [http://dx.doi.org/10.1183/09031936.00022912] [PMID: 22496332]

[15] Bolhuis MS, van Altena R, van Soolingen D, *et al.* Clarithromycin increases linezolid exposure in multidrug-resistant tuberculosis patients. Eur Respir J 2013; 42(6): 1614-21. [http://dx.doi.org/10.1183/09031936.00001913] [PMID: 23520311]

[16] The use of bedaquiline in the treatment of multidrug-resistant tuberculosis: interim policy guidance. World Health Organization 2013. WHO/HTM/TB/2013.6. ISBN 978 92 4 150548 2

[17] Skripconoka V, Danilovits M, Pehme L, *et al.* Delamanid improves outcomes and reduces mortality in multidrug-resistant tuberculosis. Eur Respir J 2013; 41(6): 1393-400. [http://dx.doi.org/10.1183/09031936.00125812] [PMID: 23018916]

[18] Gler MT, Skripconoka V, Sanchez-Garavito E, *et al.* Delamanid for multidrug-resistant pulmonary tuberculosis. N Engl J Med 2012; 366(23): 2151-60. [http://dx.doi.org/10.1056/NEJMoa1112433] [PMID: 22670901]

[19] Peloquin CA. Therapeutic drug monitoring in the treatment of tuberculosis. Drugs 2002; 62(15): 2169-83. [http://dx.doi.org/10.2165/00003495-200262150-00001] [PMID: 12381217]

CHAPTER 7

Treatment of Drug Resistant Tuberculosis

Abstract: This chapter covers the strategies recommended to build an effective regimen for drug resistant tuberculosis. Treatment outcomes for multidrug resistant tuberculosis (MDR-TB) and beyond show a progressively lower cure rate as the resistance pattern became more complex. Basically all treatment recommendations for drug-resistant tuberculosis are based on expert opinion, with just a few available clinical trials. Rifampin is the most important drug in the first line regimen; if the strain is resistant is considered as pre-MDR TB and the patient must be treated for at least 18 months. There are two types of MDR-TB patients: patients who have never been treated for tuberculosis in the past and that were infected with an already resistant strain and patients previously treated for tuberculosis. The latter are much more frequent and more difficult to treat. To design a regimen for MDR-TB the following order is recommended: include ethambutol and/or pyrazinamide (WHO recommends the use of pyrazinamide regardless of the results of the drug susceptibility testing); however this drugs should not be counted as effective drugs. As a second step, a second line injectable (amikacin, kanamycin or capreomycin) will be included. Then add a fluoroquinolone (levofloxacin or moxifloxacin). Finally to complete the regimen add as many drugs from Group 4 (ethionamide, cycloserine and PAS) as needed. If necessary, include drugs from group 5. The first choice will be linezolid.

Keywords: Amikacin, Bedaquiline, Capreomycin, Clofazimine, Cycloserine, Delamanid, Drug-resistant, Ethambutol, Ethionamide, Fluoroquinolones, Kanamycin, Linezolid, Meropenem, New cases, PAS, Previously treated, Pyrazinamide, Treatment, Tuberculosis.

INTRODUCTION

A recent meta-analysis of treatment outcomes for MDR-TB and beyond, that included over 7,000 patients from 26 treatment centers showed a progressively lower cure rate as the resistance pattern became more complex. The treatment success rate progressively decreased from 64% for patients with MDR-TB without additional resistance, to 56% for MDR-TB+resistance to an SL injectable *only*, to 48% for MDR+resistance to a fluoroquinolone *only* and to 40% for XDR-

Rafael Laniado-Laborín

TB [1].

When to suspect drug resistance in a patient with tuberculosis [2 - 4]:

1. Patients who are failing while under treatment (viable microorganisms in culture after four months of directly observed therapy (DOT)
2. Presence of positive cultures after the patient had converted his/her sputum cultures
3. Patients with bacteriologically proven relapse (especially if the patient was treated without supervision (with irregular drug intake being a strong possibility)
4. Patients who have migrated from regions with high prevalence of drug resistant tuberculosis
5. Chronic patients who have received multiple courses of antituberculosis drugs

A high degree of suspicion in these scenarios will allow an earlier detection and start an effective treatment in a drug resistant case which will translate into a better prognosis for the case and a faster curtailment of transmission of a drug resistant case in the community.

Progressive clinical and/or radiographic findings or persistence of positive sputum smears and cultures must raise the suspicion of drug resistance, even in a new case. If not already done, cultures and drug susceptibility (DST) tests must be ordered as soon as possible.

When the case is a relapse (patient treated in the past and discharged as cured) the possibility of drug resistance must be considered; cultures and DST must be ordered ***in every case***. A history of previous treatment (especially if it was self-administered) is one of the most important risk factors for the development of drug resistance. Patients that were treated under direct supervision (DOT) have a lower risk of harboring a drug resistant strain (but cultures must be processed ***in every case***). Factors involved in early relapses (which actually are disguised failures) include lack of adherence to treatment, inappropriate drug regimen (inadequate doses, insufficient number of drugs), malabsorption and exogenous infection with a different *M. tuberculosis* drug resistant strain. When a new case received a strong regimen under DOT, is highly likely that the relapse is due to drug susceptible mycobacteria (reactivation of latent bacteria that were not killed during treatment). In these cases, treatment with the same regimen can be started while waiting for the DST. Conversely, if treatment was not supervised and/or irregular and the patient is gravely ill, is immunosuppressed, or has central nervous system involvement, a standardized second line drug regimen should be started while waiting for the DST [2].

TREATMENT OF DRUG RESISTANT TUBERCULOSIS (TABLE 7.1)

Basically all treatment recommendations for drug-resistant tuberculosis are based on expert opinion, with just a few available clinical trials. For this reason, patients with MDR and XDR should be preferably treated by a clinician with experience in drug resistant tuberculosis [2 - 4].

Table 7.1. Drugs used in the treatment of drug resistant tuberculosis.

GROUP	DRUGS
Group 1. First line, oral drugs	Isoniazid (H), rifampin (R), Ethambutol (E), pyrazinamide (Z)
Group 2. Second line injectables	Amikacin (Am), Capreomycin (Cm), Kanamycin (Km)
Group 3. Fluoroquinolones	Ofloxacin (Ofx), Levofloxacin (Lfx), Moxifloxacin (Mfx), Gatifloxacin (Gfx)
Grupo 4. Second line oral drugs	Ethionamide (Et), Prothionamide (Pt), Cycloserine (Cs) Para-aminosalicylate (PAS)
Grupo 5: Drugs with modest to no evidence of efficacy (except for Linezolid)	Clofazimine (Cfz), Amoxicillin/Clavulanate (Amx/Clv), Clarithromycin (Clr), Linezolid (Lzd), Imipenem/Cilastatin (Imp/Cln)

TREATMENT FOR MONO-RESISTANCE [3]

Isolated Resistance to Isoniazid (H)

Patients can be treated with E-R-Z daily for 9 months; in cases with extensive disease a fluoroquinolone (Mfx/Lfx/Gfx) could be added to the regimen to substitute H (R-E- Z-FQ) in a daily regimen for at least 6 months.

Isolated Resistance to Rifampin (R)

Rifampin is the most important drug in the first line regimen; if the strain is resistant to R the case will be considered as pre-XDR TB. Patient can be treated with H+E+FQ+Et+Z for at least 18 months. In patients with extensive disease, an injectable can be added to the regimen until culture conversion. Substituting R with rifabutin is not recommended, since up to 80% of R resistant strains there is cross-resistance to rifabutin (and almost 100% to rifapentine).

Isolated Resistance to Ethambutol (E), Pyrazinamide (Z) or Streptomycin (S)

Isolated resistance to E, Z or S had very little impact on the efficacy of the regimen; for E and S it does not need any change in the regimen or its length. For Z, due to its early intracellular bactericidal effect, the follow up phase of the regimen with H and R should be extended for three extra months for a total of 9 months of treatment.

TREATMENT FOR POLYRESISTANT CASES

Resistance to Isoniazid and Pyrazinamide

Recommended regimen includes R+E+FQ at least for 9-12 months (or longer for patients with extensive disease).

Resistance to Isoniazid and Ethambutol

Recommended regimen should include R+Z+FQ at least for 9-12 months (or longer for patients with extensive disease).

Resistance to Rifampin and Ethambutol (± Streptomycin)

Regimen should include H+Z+FQ for 18 months plus a second line injectable during the first 2-3 months (or up to 6 months in patients with extensive disease.

Resistance to Rifampin and Pyrazinamide (± Streptomycin)

Recommended regimen includes I+E+FQ for 18 months plus a second line injectable during the first 2-3 months (or up to 6 months in patients with extensive disease.

Resistance to Isoniazid + Ethambutol + Pyrazinamide (± Streptomycin)

Regimen should include R+FQ + oral second line drug (cycloserine, PAS or ethionamide; this last one is not a good choice if resistance to H is only low concentration since there is high probability of cross resistance) for 18 months plus a second line injectable during the first 2-3 months (or up to 6 months in patients with extensive disease.

BUILDING A REGIMEN FOR MDR-TB [2 - 4]

Basically we are facing two types of MDR-TB patients: patients who have never been treated for tuberculosis in the past and that were infected with an already resistant strain (classified as "new cases" or "primary resistance") and patients previously treated for tuberculosis (resistance in "treated cases" or "acquired resistance"). The latter are much more frequent and more difficult to treat.

In cases with risk factors for drug resistance, the availability of a rapid diagnosis test (for example the XpertMTB/RIFA(r) system which allows detection of rifampin resistance in about two hours) would help the treating physician to select a modified regimen while waiting for the drug susceptibility testing (DST) results, instead of using the standardized first line drugs regimen that would almost certainly lead to treatment failure and amplification of drug resistance. This initial modified regimen (usually a standardized second line drug regimen) can be customized as needed when the DST results are reported. Obviously, the regimen ***must be directly observed***.

In patients with a history of antituberculosis treatment, the presence of drug resistance is invariably iatrogenic, including unsupervised treatment with lack of adherence, inadequate drug regimens or drug doses, not detecting primary resistance in a new case, *etc*.

In a true relapse (*e.g.* a patient that completed DOT, discharged as cured with negative sputum smears/cultures and later on develops clinical disease and bacteriologic relapse), the causing strain is almost always due to drug susceptible latent mycobacteria that were not eradicated during treatment, and as a result of its low or null multiplication rate it is highly unlikely that they will develop spontaneous drug resistant mutants. These patients can be treated with first line drugs while waiting for the DST results. Although the probability of having a drug resistant strain is low, all relapse cases should have samples sent for culture and

DST.

Treatment failure is due to mycobacteria that are actively reproducing, generating spontaneous mutations that can confer resistance to antituberculosis drugs, creating favorable conditions for the selection of these resistant bacteria. A high proportion of cases with treatment failure will harbor drug-resistant mycobacteria and probably include resistant mutations for every drug in the regimen. ***Culture and DST must be carried out in every single case of treatment failure***. If the patient is failing treatment while under direct supervision, serum drug levels should be obtained, if testing is available, to rule out the possibility of malabsorption as the cause of treatment failure.

Another important group of patients with high risk of drug resistance is that of patients who have defaulted treatment. When a patient abandons treatment stopping all drugs at the same time (more likely when multiple drugs are included in one pill) the risk of selecting resistant mutants is lower than that of patients that is receiving multiple individual drugs and stop taking some of the drugs (usually due to some type of side effect that the patient attributes to that drug, whether this is real or not) but continue taking others. In this situation, the probability of selecting resistant mutants is very high with the consequent amplification of drug resistance.

Another frequent scenario is that of patients with poor adherence to treatment, with irregular intake of the antituberculosis drugs while under self-administered treatment. This could be easily avoided with DOT. This is more frequent during the final phase of treatment, when the patient is usually asymptomatic and still has to continue receiving treatment. When this irregular intake of antituberculosis drugs linger for weeks or months, conditions are created for selecting resistant mutants. It's important to take into account that the post-antibiotic effect (time period during which the antibiotic is still effective after one dose) of drugs included in the regimen is extremely variable. For example, the post-antibiotic effect of isoniazid is much longer than that of rifampin; if the patient is receiving H+R three time a week during the final 4 months of treatment, and fails to receive one of the doses, the post-antibiotic effect of H will be longer than that of R and the patient will be inadvertently under monotherapy with H during a couple of days. If this pattern of irregular intake of drugs persist it favors the selection of H resistant mutations and later on of R resistant mutations. The most difficult therapeutic challenge however is that of patients with chronic tuberculosis that have received several courses of treatment over the years, including empiric regimens containing fluoroquinolones and/or second line injectables. The clinician must have in these cases a high degree of suspicion of the presence of a strain resistant to multiple drugs. It is extremely important to obtain a careful pharmacological history of drugs received by the patient in previous regimens (verifying it from the patient's files if available) and obtain DST not only for first line drugs but also for second line drugs, especially for quinolones and second line injectable. Is necessary to go over treatment history with as much detail as possible to ascertain when a drug was started and was stopped, doses, drugs that were administered simultaneously.

Due to the multiple possible patterns of resistance there are very few clinical trials or evidence based recommendations and most of the treatment recommendations in MDR-TB are based on expert opinion. Some basic principles however, are time tested and should be considered when building a treatment regimen for MDR-TB case:

1. Combine the information obtained in the pharmacological history and the results from the DST (it is assumed that testing was done in a reliable laboratory)
2. Combine 4 (and preferably 5) drugs that have never been used by the patient or are shown to still be effective on DST
3. Ideally, the regimen should be structured in consultation with an expert on drug resistant tuberculosis

To design a regimen the following order is recommended:

1. Include those first line drugs (basically E) that according to DST it still remain effective; the WHO recommends the addition of Z to every MDR-TB treatment regimen based on the low reliability of DST for this drug; however both drugs (E and Z) should not be counted as effective drugs.
2. As a second step, a second line injectable (Group **2:** Amk, Km or Cm); DST for these drugs are very reliable. Resistance to S does not usually present cross resistance with second line injectables. Resistance to injectable drugs is considered as unidirectional and is recommended to use Km initially; if a resistant mutation to Km appears during

treatment, Cm and Amk will usually still be active; conversely resistance to Amk will frequently be associated to cross resistance to Km and Cm.

3. Add a fluoroquinolone (**Group 3**: Lfx, Mfx,Gfx). DST for these drugs are very reliable.
4. Finally to complete the regimen add as many drugs from Group 4 (oral bacteriostatic drugs: Eth/Pth, Cs or PAS) as needed, based on pharmacological history and DST (however take into account that DST for group 4 drugs are not reliable and/or reproducible).
5. If a 4-5 drugs regimen cannot be completed so far, it will necessary to include drugs from group 5. The first choice will be Lzn that has proven efficacy, but toxicity and cost limit its use. For the other drugs from this group (clofazimine, amoxicillin/clavulanate, imipenem/meropenem, macrolides) there is little evidence of efficacy and they are included when there is no other choice.

Injectable is administered 5-7 times per week, either by the intramuscular (IM) or intravenous (IV) route through a central catheter. Once the patient becomes culture negative it can be spaced to 3 times per week. Traditionally the injectable is maintained at least for six months after culture conversion in patients with extensive disease, slow microbiologic response or very complex resistance pattern.

When selecting drugs is necessary to consider the possibility of cross-resistance between antituberculosis drugs (Table **7.2**):

Table 7.2. Cross resistance among antituberculosis drugs.

DRUG	CROSS-RESISTANCE	COMMENT
Isoniazid	Ethionamide	When low grade resistance to H is present
Rifampin	Rifamycins	Cross resistance with rifabutin and rifapentine is common
Ethambutol, Pyrazinamide & Streptomycin	None	
Amikacin	Kanamycin	High probability since its due to the same mutation
Capreomycin	None	
Fluoroquinolones	Other fluoroquinolones	Resistance to one FQ is not necessarily associated to cross resistance to other FQ
Cycloserine	None	

(Table 7.1) contd.....

DRUG	CROSS-RESISTANCE	COMMENT
PAS	None	

It is well known that when a patient has used a drug for more than a month, there is a possibility that drug might not be effective, even when the DST show that there is no resistance, especially in the case of E and Z. If these drugs are included in the regimen they should not be considered as one of the 4-5 effective drugs ("include them but do not count them").

Practical Aspects of Multidrug Resistant Tuberculosis Treatment

Success rates of treatment for drug resistant TB are much lower than those for susceptible TB, and the higher the resistance the lower the success rate. Treatment success for pan susceptible TB under DOT can be as high as 95%, while it is only 64% for MDR-TB, 56% for MDR-TB plus resistance to a second line injectable (SLI), 48% for MDR-TB plus resistance to a fluoroquinolone, 40-43% for XDR, 34% for XDR with resistance to all SLI and 19% for XDR+all SLI+E+Z [5].

It is vital to emphasize that ***all patients with drug resistant TB must be under strict DOT*** under the supervision of health personnel with experience in the treatment of DR-TB. Unlike first line drugs that are administered all together once a day (especially when multidrug tablets are available), second line drugs are available only on individual presentation and frequently the daily dose must be divided in two to lessen side effects (*e.g.* PAS, ethionamide, cycloserine) and this could lead to selective lack of adherence if unsupervised.

To reduce the impact of side effects and the probability of the patient defaulting treatment, it is recommended to start with a half the dose of ethionamide, cycloserine and PAS and ramp up to the full dose within a couple of weeks.

Length of treatment for MDR-TB will depend on several factors that include what drugs are included in the regimen, extent of disease and especially time needed for definite culture conversion. In general minimum duration is 18 months post culture conversion (regardless of when treatment was started) and in some cases up to 24 months.

Regarding MDR, remember...

1. Complexity of treatment for MDR-TB requires that it should be carried out exclusively by expert personnel. Unfortunately, in countries with the highest rates of MDR-TB there are not enough experts available to supervise all cases
2. Never add a single drug to a failing treatment regimen. Add as many bactericidal drugs as possible with different mycobacterial target
3. Include at least 4 drugs that have never been used by the patient in the past and for which DST have shown efficacy
4. Sufficient number of oral drugs must be included in the regimen for it to be strong enough when the injectable is stopped
5. Without exception, treatment must always be DOT
6. Intermittent regimens are never used for MDR-TB (except for second line injectables that can be spaced after culture conversion)
7. It is not recommended to use drugs for which DST show resistance; in general they will have null clinical efficacy. Treatment of an MDR-TB case might be the last opportunity for a patient to be cured, and the best available drug regimen must be used every time
8. There is no cross resistance between S and Km/Amk, but cross resistance between Am and Km is virtually universal

Surgery for Patients with Drug Resistant TB

Surgery has a very limited role in the treatment of drug resistant TB. Some experts suggest that patients with positive cultures after 4-6 months of treatment and/or with such an extensive resistance pattern that it makes it improbable to attain culture conversion exclusively with drug treatment, should undergo resectional surgery [6].

A recent meta-analysis on surgical treatment for MDR-TB and XDR-TB that included 24 studies published from 1975 through 2012 reported a significant association between surgical treatment and successful outcome in comparison with non-surgical treatment (OR of favorable outcome 2.24, 95%CI 1.68-2.97). Benefit from surgery was directly related to increasing drug resistance [7].

However, this view is not shared by most experts in the field, since there is insufficient evidence to recommend surgery plus chemotherapy over chemotherapy alone. To be a surgical candidate, the patient must have limited disease, enough functional reserve to tolerate a lobectomy or pneumonectomy, in general have an acceptable surgical risk and enough drugs left to structure an effective regimen to avoid late complications of surgery.

Unfortunately most chronic MDR-TB patients will not satisfy this criteria, especially since most will have extensive bilateral disease with very limited functional reserve. Of course if surgery is an option it must be performed by an experience surgeon in a hospital that has the infrastructure to offer adequate postoperative care. Even if surgery is successful, medical treatment must be continued for at least 18-24 months.

SHORT COURSE TREATMENT FOR MDR-TB: THE "BANGLADESH REGIMEN"

As already mentioned, treatment regimens for MDR-TB are very long, often poorly tolerated, and difficult to monitor. A project to test a short course regimen for drug resistant TB was conducted by the tuberculosis services of the Damien Foundation in Bangladesh, a nongovernmental organization implementing tuberculosis services in close collaboration with the government. Six different regimens were used with a 9-month regimen (4 months intensive phase of Km, Clf, Gfx, E, H (high dose), Z, Pth followed by a 5 month continuation phase of Gfx, E, Z, Clf) being the most effective with a relapse free cure of 87.9% among 206 patients. It is important to mention that patients that had received second line drugs for as long as one month were excluded from the study [8]. There urgent need to determine through more extensive clinical trials under different conditions, if these results can be replicated.

Individualized or Standardized Treatment [9]?

In everyday practice, we are frequently faced by a chronic patient that has been treated repeatedly with first line drugs and is still symptomatic and smear positive. Obviously, we have a high suspicion of multidrug resistance and we will have to decide which type of regimen would be the most effective: a second line drug standardized empiric regimen (based on the patterns of drug resistance in the region) without the benefit of DST, or individualized regimen that combines the information from the pharmacological history and the results from the DST. The choice usually depends on access to rapid diagnosis tests (GeneXpertMTB/RIF®, GenoType-MTBDRplus®) and availability of second line drugs.

We need to start treatment as soon as possible to reduce the morbidity (and mortality) of the individual patient and to stop the chain of transmission of a resistant strain in the community. Although the combination of pharmacological history and results from the DST (including those for second line drugs) allows for the selection of an individually tailored regimen, DST reports (especially for second line drugs) can be delayed for months. The best solution for this type of cases is to start with a standardized second line drug regimen that includes at least 4-5 drugs that the patient has never received in the past (with a fluoroquinolone, a SL injectable and ethionamide/prothionamide as a backbone). This regimen then can be modified when receiving the results from the DST.

WHO GUIDELINES FOR THE PROGRAMMATIC MANAGEMENT OF DRUG-RESISTANT TUBERCULOSIS – 2011 UPDATE [4]

In its latest update (2011) on treatment for MDR-TB the World Health Organization recommends to always include a fluoroquinolone (Lfx, Mfx or Gfx; ciprofloxacin and ofloxacin should not be use any more) ethionamide/prothionamide. a second line injectable, pyrazinamide (regardless of the DST results), cycloserine and/or PAS. According to the WHO guideline, a regimen built with drugs that have shown efficacy on DST have only a marginal benefit in comparison to a standardized regimen that does not take into account the results from the DST. The argument for this position is based on the poor reproducibility of DST for pyrazinamide and for the second line drugs (except for fluoroquinolones and second line injectables). However, the same document mentions that the use of a recent generation fluoroquinolone is associated with a better prognosis, especially if the DST shows susceptibility to the drug. Since there are no clear advantage among the second line injectables, kanamycin is recommended due to its lower cost. Streptomycin is not recommended for patient with MDR-TB. Ethionamide is considered more effective than cycloserine, which in turn is considered more effective than PAS. This last drug is only recommended when a 5th drug is needed to complete the regimen or when there is resistance to ethionamide. There is no evidence to determine if PAS should be administered in one or two doses. The decision will depend on the patientA's tolerance and available resources for DOT. The WHO states that there is no evidence of the efficacy of group 5 drugs amoxicillin/clavulanate, clofazimine, macrolides and thioacetazone and the experience with INH at high doses, pyrazinamide, ethambutol and linezolid is not enough to issue a recommendation. Finally the document states that the use of additional drugs in patients with extensive disease has no supporting evidence in the literature.

It is important to emphasize that the guideline states that this recommendations have very little supporting evidence, and are mostly based on expert opinion.

Some experts [10] consider that clofazimine may contribute to new short-course MDR-TB regimens (like the Bangladesh regimen), and the beta-lactams (imipenem, meropenem) merit further evaluation [11].

Linezolid is very effective but its use is limited by cost and frequent side effects. *Mycobacterium tuberculosis* has intrinsic inducible resistance to clarithromycin and its only contribution to a treatment regimen is to increase the serum levels of linezolid, which allows using a lower (and less costly) dose of this drug [12].

EXTENSIVELY DRUG RESISTANT TUBERCULOSIS

Patients who harbor an extensively drug resistant strain are left with less available effective drugs, and frequently the regimen must include less potent and more toxic drugs for which there is little evidence of their efficacy [13]. Currently, XDR-TB is defined as MDR-TB plus resistance to fluoroquinolones and to at least to one of the second-line (SL) injectables (kanamycin, amikacin and capreomycin). There is controversy about this definition, because although in general it carries an ominous prognosis, it might not be so in all cases [14]. Some strains can present mutations that confer resistance to one fluoroquinolone but not to others and the same can occur for SL injectables. These patients can then be treated with a regimen that includes an effective fluoroquinolone and SL injectable and may consequently have a prognosis that is very close to that of MDR-TB. A better definition of XDR-TB would be for those strains that are MDR and also resistant to all fluoroquinolones and all SL injectables.

Systematic revisions show that success rates for treatment of XDR-TB are very low (less than 50% defined as cure plus treatment completion) and mortality rates extremely high (more than 20%) [15].

It seems logical that the optimal number of drugs included in the treatment for XDR-TB should be higher than those recommended for MDR-TB. A recent meta-analysis showed that the use of at least six drugs during the intensive phase and at least four effective drugs during the continuation phase was associated with better treatment success [1].

Regarding the duration of treatment, the highest treatment success rates were observed when treatment was prolonged for a total duration of up to 18-25 months [1, 16].

There is not enough evidence to establish the importance of individual drugs in the treatment of XDR-TB. For example, even though resistance to fluoroquinolones is part of the definition of XDR-TB, incomplete cross resistance between this class of drugs may explain why the use of a FQ in XDR-TB, even when DST reveal resistance to a representative FQ, significantly improves treatment outcomes [1, 13].

Linezolid (LNZ) is without a doubt the most important drug in the treatment of XDR-TB, especially if the strain is resistant to all available fluoroquinolones. A systematic review and meta-analysis that included 121 patients from 12 studies reported a treatment success rate of 82% [17]. In a clinical trial LNZ (600 mg daily PO) was added to the background regimen at the start of treatment and compared with the control group which added LNZ after two months of treatment. The primary end point was the time to sputum-culture conversion at 4 months culture conversion was achieved in 79% of patients that received LNZ from the start *vs*. 35% of those who did not ($p < 0.001$). Overall, 87% of the patients had a negative sputum culture within 6 months after linezolid had been added to their drug regimen [18]. The most important limitations of LNZ are its cost (about $60 US dollars per 600 mg tablet) and its toxicity. Although there is a report of an inexpensive and effective presentation of LNZ (less than $1 US dollar), this is only available in India [19]. Most serious toxicity include myelossupression and neuropathy which are directly related to dose and length of treatment [13].

Clofazimine is a rediscovered compound in group 5 that has been used for many years in the treatment of leprosy. Its efficacy has been tested in MDR [8] and it can be a useful drug as part of a regimen for treatment of XDR-TB according to a systematic review and meta-analysis [20]; its toxicity (skin pigmentation, icthyosis, rash, gastrointestinal intolerance) seems to be less severe than that of other second line drugs.

Carbapenems (combined with clavulanate) at high doses have shown efficacy when combined with linezolid containing regimen in MDR cases. In a clinical trial including MDR & XDR TB patients, the group receiving meropenem-clavulanate+linezolid (plus the WHO recommended regimen) had an 83.8% culture conversion rate *vs.* 62.5% the controls, although this difference did not reach statistical difference (p=0.06). When the XDR-cases were excluded from the analysis, this difference did reach statistical significance [21].

The WHO has recommended the addition of bedaquiline to a WHO approved regimen in adult MDR-TB patients when there is also evidence of resistance to any fluoroquinolone (what is known as pre-XDRTB) [21]. This recommendation is based on very weak evidence, since bedaquiline was approved by the FDA after being tested in only two clinical trials that included 208 patients [22, 23]. Bedaquiline has important safety concerns (it prolongs the Q-T interval, and effect that can be additive if used concomitantly with delamanid or fluoroquinolones). Also a higher mortality rate was reported in the group treated with bedaquiline compared with placebo [24].

Delamanid has been tested on MDR-TB patients in combination with a background regimen developed according to the WHO guidelines; the delamanid group had significantly higher rate of sputum culture-conversion rate at 2 months than that of the control group [25].

In another report [26] assessing the outcome in a subset of XDR-TB patients treated with delamanid (outcomes were defined as favorable if patients were cured or completed treatment or unfavorable if failed, died or defaulted) there was higher proportion of favorable outcomes after extended treatment with delamanid

(61.4% *vs*. 50.0% for the control group); all patients with XDR-TB who had received delamanid for at least 6 months survived.

CONFLICT OF INTEREST

The author confirms that this chapter has no conflict of interest.

ACKNOWLEDGEMENTS

None declared.

REFERENCES

[1] Falzon D, Gandhi N, Migliori GB, *et al.* Collaborative Group for Meta-Analysis of Individual Patient Data in MDR-TB. Resistance to fluoroquinolones and second-line injectable drugs: impact on multidrug-resistant TB outcomes. Eur Respir J 2013; 42(1): 156-68. [http://dx.doi.org/10.1183/09031936.00134712] [PMID: 23100499]

[2] Caminero JA. Management of multidrug-resistant tuberculosis and patients in retreatment. Eur Respir J 2005; 25(5): 928-36. [http://dx.doi.org/10.1183/09031936.05.00103004] [PMID: 15863653]

[3] Curry International Tuberculosis Center and California Department of Public Health. Drug-Resistant Tuberculosis: A Survival Guide for Clinicians. (2nd ed.), 2011.

[4] Guidelines for the programmatic management of drug-resistant tuberculosis – 2011 update. World Health Organization 2011. ISBN 9789241501583

[5] Caminero JA, Matteelli A, Loddenkemper R. Tuberculosis: are we making it incurable? Eur Respir J 2013; 42(1): 5-8. [http://dx.doi.org/10.1183/09031936.00206712] [PMID: 23813308]

[6] Goble M, Iseman MD, Madsen LA, Waite D, Ackerson L, Horsburgh CR Jr. Treatment of 171 patients with pulmonary tuberculosis resistant to isoniazid and rifampin. N Engl J Med 1993; 328(8): 527-32. [http://dx.doi.org/10.1056/NEJM199302253280802] [PMID: 8426619]

[7] Marrone MT, Venkataramanan V, Goodman M, Hill AC, Jereb JA, Mase SR. Surgical interventions for drug-resistant tuberculosis: a systematic review and meta-analysis. Int J Tuberc Lung Dis 2013; 17(1): 6-16. [http://dx.doi.org/10.5588/ijtld.12.0198] [PMID: 23232000]

[8] Aung KJ, Van Deun A, Declercq E, *et al.* Successful '9-month Bangladesh regimen' for multidrug-resistant tuberculosis among over 500 consecutive patients. Int J Tuberc Lung Dis 2014; 18(10): 1180-7. [http://dx.doi.org/10.5588/ijtld.14.0100] [PMID: 25216831]

[9] Laniado-LaborA-n R. Multidrug-resistant tuberculosis: standardized or individualized treatment? The question has already been answered. Expert Rev Respir Med 2010; 4(2): 143-6. [http://dx.doi.org/10.1586/ers.10.6] [PMID: 20406077]

[10] Dooley KE, Obuku EA, Durakovic N, Belitsky V, Mitnick C, Nuermberger EL. Efficacy Subgroup, RESIST-TB. World Health Organization group 5 drugs for the treatment of drug-resistant tuberculosis: unclear efficacy or untapped potential? J Infect Dis 2013; 207(9): 1352-8.
[http://dx.doi.org/10.1093/infdis/jis460] [PMID: 22807518]

[11] Cholo MC, Steel HC, Fourie PB, Germishuizen WA, Anderson R. Clofazimine: current status and future prospects. J Antimicrob Chemother 2012; 67(2): 290-8.
[http://dx.doi.org/10.1093/jac/dkr444] [PMID: 22020137]

[12] Bolhuis MS, van Altena R, Uges DR, van der Werf TS, Kosterink JG, Alffenaar JW. Clarithromycin significantly increases linezolid serum concentrations. Antimicrob Agents Chemother 2010; 54(12): 5418-9.
[http://dx.doi.org/10.1128/AAC.00757-10] [PMID: 20837753]

[13] Matteelli A, Roggi A, Carvalho AC. Extensively drug-resistant tuberculosis: epidemiology and management. Clin Epidemiol 2014; 6: 111-8.
[http://dx.doi.org/10.2147/CLEP.S35839] [PMID: 24729727]

[14] Caminero JA. Extensively drug-resistant tuberculosis: is its definition correct? Eur Respir J 2008; 32(5): 1413-5. [Letter].
[http://dx.doi.org/10.1183/09031936.00094708] [PMID: 18978145]

[15] Jacobson KR, Tierney DB, Jeon CY, Mitnick CD, Murray MB. Treatment outcomes among patients with extensively drug-resistant tuberculosis: systematic review and meta-analysis. Clin Infect Dis 2010; 51(1): 6-14.
[http://dx.doi.org/10.1086/653115] [PMID: 20504231]

[16] Migliori GB, Sotgiu G, Gandhi NR, *et al.* Drug resistance beyond XDR-TB: results from a large individual patient data meta-analysis. Eur Respir J 2013; 42: 169-79.
[http://dx.doi.org/10.1183/09031936.00136312] [PMID: 23060633]

[17] Sotgiu G, Centis R, D'Ambrosio L, *et al.* Efficacy, safety and tolerability of linezolid containing regimens in treating MDR-TB and XDR-TB: systematic review and meta-analysis. Eur Respir J 2012; 40(6): 1430-42.
[http://dx.doi.org/10.1183/09031936.00022912] [PMID: 22496332]

[18] Lee M, Lee J, Carroll MW, *et al.* Linezolid for treatment of chronic extensively drug-resistant tuberculosis. N Engl J Med 2012; 367(16): 1508-18.
[http://dx.doi.org/10.1056/NEJMoa1201964] [PMID: 23075177]

[19] Singla R, Caminero JA, Jaiswal A, *et al.* Linezolid: an effective, safe and cheap drug for patients failing multidrug-resistant tuberculosis treatment in India. Eur Respir J 2012; 39(4): 956-62.
[http://dx.doi.org/10.1183/09031936.00076811] [PMID: 21965225]

[20] Dey T, Brigden G, Cox H, Shubber Z, Cooke G, Ford N. Outcomes of clofazimine for the treatment of drug-resistant tuberculosis: a systematic review and meta-analysis. J Antimicrob Chemother 2013; 68(2): 284-93.
[http://dx.doi.org/10.1093/jac/dks389] [PMID: 23054996]

[21] De Lorenzo S, Alffenaar JW, Sotgiu G, *et al.* Efficacy and safety of meropenem-clavulanate added to linezolid-containing regimens in the treatment of MDR-/XDR-TB. Eur Respir J 2013; 41(6): 1386-92.

[http://dx.doi.org/10.1183/09031936.00124312] [PMID: 22997218]

[22] Diacon AH, Pym A, Grobusch M, *et al.* The diarylquinoline TMC207 for multidrug-resistant tuberculosis. N Engl J Med 2009; 360(23): 2397-405.
[http://dx.doi.org/10.1056/NEJMoa0808427] [PMID: 19494215]

[23] Diacon AH, Donald PR, Pym A, *et al.* Randomized pilot trial of eight weeks of bedaquiline (TMC207) treatment for multidrug-resistant tuberculosis: long-term outcome, tolerability, and effect on emergence of drug resistance. Antimicrob Agents Chemother 2012; 56(6): 3271-6.
[http://dx.doi.org/10.1128/AAC.06126-11] [PMID: 22391540]

[24] World Health Organization. The Use of Bedaquiline in the Treatment of Multidrug-Resistant Tuberculosis: Interim Policy Guidance. Geneva: WHO 2013.

[25] Gler MT, Skripconoka V, Sanchez-Garavito E, *et al.* Delamanid for multidrug-resistant pulmonary tuberculosis. N Engl J Med 2012; 366(23): 2151-60.
[http://dx.doi.org/10.1056/NEJMoa1112433] [PMID: 22670901]

[26] Skripconoka V, Danilovits M, Pehme L, *et al.* Delamanid improves outcomes and reduces mortality in multidrug-resistant tuberculosis. Eur Respir J 2013; 41(6): 1393-400.
[http://dx.doi.org/10.1183/09031936.00125812] [PMID: 23018916]

CHAPTER 8

Adverse Effects and Toxicity of Antituberculosis Drugs

Abstract: This chapter covers side and adverse effects associated to antituberculosis treatment. Gastrointestinal side effects are usually the first to appear after the start of treatment, with nausea and vomiting being the most common. Drug regimens for multidrug resistant tuberculosis include drugs that very frequently produce side effects and/or toxicity that sometimes require the definitive suspension of the drug. Almost all patients undergoing drug treatment for MDR-TB experience some type of side effects and/or toxicity that involve a modification of the drug regimen in up to 50% of the cases. A problem associated to second-line drugs is that several of these drugs share side effects and toxicities, which makes it difficult sometimes to determine which drug is the culprit. It is extremely important to avoid as much as possible interruptions in treatment due to side effects because this decreases the effectiveness of the regimen and increases the risk of amplifying drug resistance. Peripheral neuropathy is more common in patients that are already prone to it such as diabetics, alcoholics, pregnant and malnourished patients. All antituberculosis injectable drugs are toxic to the eight cranial nerve and can cause both vestibular (equilibrium) and cochlear (auditory) damage. Hepatic toxicity is the most common adverse effect of antituberculosis treatment and its severity can range from asymptomatic elevation of liver enzymes to fulminant liver insufficiency with encephalopathy and high mortality. Although any patient under treatment with antituberculosis drugs can develop hepatic toxicity, patients with previous liver damage are at higher risk of this complication.

Keywords: Adverse, Ataxia, Creatinine, Effects, Enzymes, Hepatotoxicity, Hypersensitivity, Liver, MDR-TB, Neuropathy, Renal failure, Stevens-Johnson, Toxicity, Optic neuritis, Urticaria, Vestibular, Vertigo.

INTRODUCTION

Patients undergoing treatment for pan-sensitive tuberculosis usually tolerate the drug regimen without any significant side effect or toxicity, and when they do, these are usually moderate and transient. Quite the opposite, drug regimens for multidrug resistant tuberculosis include drugs that very frequently produce side

Rafael Laniado-Laborín

effects and/or toxicity that sometimes require the definitive suspension of the drug.

The true frequency of these side effects is unknown because they are usually not notified by the treating physician and thus are not reported. Clinical experience shows that almost all patients undergoing drug treatment for MDR-TB experience some type of side effects and/or toxicity that involve a modification of the drug regimen in up to 50% of the cases.

A problem associated to second-line drugs is that several of these drugs share side effects and toxicities, which makes it difficult sometimes to determine which drug is the culprit. Although the frequency of very severe side effects is low, in some cases they can be life-threatening, including anaphylactic reactions, Stevens-Johnson syndrome and erosive gastritis with gastrointestinal bleeding, fulminant hepatitis and renal failure.

When a patient has an adverse effect during treatment, the first step will be to verify if the drug doses are correct for the patient´s age, weight and special characteristics (diabetic, renal disease, *etc.*); it is vital to rule out that the symptoms are not due to other causes; for example in a patient developing hepatitis, this could be due to a viral infection and not necessarily associated to drug regimen.

It must be discussed with the patient what are the benefits and risks of treating MDR-TB and the need to include several drugs to integrate an effective regimen. It is very important to explain at the onset of treatment, what side effects and toxicity can be associated to the drugs included in the regimen, and also, our limited margin for modifying the drug scheme, with the purpose of achieving their cooperation and tolerance to avoid modification of the regimen when minor side effects are present. The patient must be fully aware that this might be the last opportunity to be cured, and if they default treatment, the next regimen (if there is still an option for an effective scheme) will be more toxic and less effective. They must be assured that every effort will be made to minimize the side effects associated to treatment by adding ancillary drugs for nausea, polyneuritis, heartburn, *etc.*

It is extremely important to avoid as much as possible interruptions in treatment due to side effects because this decreases the effectiveness of the regimen and increases the risk of amplifying drug resistance. We must pay attention to side effects, actively evaluating them at each visit. Most patients are willing to tolerate minor side effects if we reassure them that a certain side effect is not serious and will not produce sequelae.

To minimize the impact of side and adverse effects on treatment adherence it is vital that health personnel is adequately trained and experienced to be able to diagnose and treat complications as soon as they appear. Standardized protocols and ancillary drugs to treat side effects must be in place and available in all tuberculosis programs.

ADVERSE EFFECTS AND TOXICITY [1 - 4]

Hypersensitivity And Cutaneous Reactions

Hypersensitivity. Virtually all antituberculosis drugs can in theory produce a hypersensitivity reaction. If severe, this type of reaction requires in general stopping all drugs until the reaction subsides. Isoniazid, ethambutol, rifampin pyrazinamide, ethionamide and the fluoroquinolones are the more frequently involved. If the reaction is mild and there is no evidence of anaphylaxis, angioedema or respiratory distress, we can try to identify the responsible drug by reintroducing the drug one at a time; it is recommended to start with the most important drug of the regimen, unless that for some reasons that is the suspect drug. Re-challenge with progressively higher doses can be tried as long as the drug is tolerated; for example, the drug can be re-started at $1/10^{th}$ of its original dose, and then if tolerated, increase the drug progressively to its full dose within a week. If the reaction was severe, the challenge must be conducted with the patient hospitalized to be able to immediately treat an anaphylactic reaction. If the drugs are reintroduced without an adverse reaction, the regimen must be then administered 7 days a week including Sundays, since hypersensitivity reactions are seen more frequently during intermittent treatment. If the patient has an anaphylactic reaction or the reaction included systemic manifestations (fever, urticaria, Stevens-Johnson syndrome) re-challenge is contraindicated and a different regimen must be utilized.

Pruritus and Maculopapular Rash

These are frequent effects that usually resolve after a few weeks without the need of interrupting treatment. If the pruritus is mild it can be treated with an antihistaminic drug; in more severe cases an oral steroid at low doses (*e.g.* prednisone 10-20 mg/day) can be used. Other causes of dermatitis such as scabies, contact dermatitis, atopic dermatitis, psoriasis, *etc.* must be considered. Dry skin in diabetics can cause pruritus. Clofazimine can cause severe dryness of the skin.

Photosensitivity can be caused by pyrazinamide, fluoroquinolones and especially by clofazimine. Clofazimine produces orange to brownish skin pigmentation as similar discoloration of most bodily fluids and secretions. These discolorations are reversible but may take months to years to disappear. Cases of icthyosis and skin dryness have also been reported in response to clofazimine (8–28%). Hyper-pigmentation of the skin associated with the use of clofazimine can aggravated with direct exposure to sunlight. Patients must be warned to avoid sunlight as much as possible, and to protect their skin with sunscreen [5].

Lichenoid Reactions

They occasionally appear in the wrists, shins or back as pruritic violaceous papules. They can resolve spontaneously; if persistent they can be treated with an antihistaminic or low dose prednisone. It is difficult to pinpoint the offending drugs since this type of reaction has been described with several of the antituberculosis drugs.

PERIPHERAL NEUROPATHY

Polyneuropathy due to antituberculosis drugs is a frequent side effect manifested by peripheral tingling, numbness, pruritus and burning sensation on the soles or toes. If progressive, it will produce sensory loss and loss of tendon reflexes, with balance disorders due to proprioceptive compromise.

Peripheral neuropathy is more common in patients that are already prone to it such as diabetics, alcoholics, pregnant and malnourished patients.

Diagnosis is based on clinical symptoms. Neuropathy is more frequently caused by isoniazid, ethionamide, cycloserine and linezolid [6]. Ethambutol and the fluoroquinolones can occasionally produce peripheral neuropathy.

To prevent these side effect patients on regimens that include ethionamide, cycloserine, linezolid or isoniazid at high doses should receive 100 mg of pyridoxine (B6). In severe cases, neuropathy can be treated with carbamazepine or gabapentin.

CENTRAL NERVOUS SYSTEM SIDE EFFECTS

Somnolence, headaches and anxiety are common in the initial phases of treatment; they are usually mild and resolve spontaneously without the need of interrupting the regimen.

Depression is also common if the regimen includes isoniazid, ethionamide and especially cycloserine. Usually it is mild and does not require specific treatment. It's important to consider that these patients are frequently depressed due to their chronic disease, and in part due to their loss of trust on the health system that have failed to cure them in the past. It is very important to regain the patient´s trust in this new drug regimen if we hope that the patient will adhere to a treatment that could extend for two or more years. If needed, we should seek psychological support. If the patient is going to be treated with antidepressants we must be aware of possible drug interactions; for example, if a patient is being treated with linezolid tricyclic antidepressants are contraindicated. If clinical depression is severe at the start of treatment cycloserine should not be included in the drug regimen. Cycloserine can induce psychotic episodes and suicidal ideation; in this scenario cycloserine should be stopped immediately. Other drugs that can induce a psychotic crisis are fluoroquinolones and isoniazid, although for both drugs this occurs infrequently. If available, serum levels of the drugs should be obtained to assure that the levels are within therapeutic range.

Seizures are a serious complication of drug treatment that requires hospitalization; they can be secondary to pyridoxine depletion and will require intravenous administration of B6. The causative drug must be stopped (usually cycloserine, fluoroquinolones or isoniazid) and anticonvulsive treatment should be started immediately and continued for as long as the patient is receiving treatment for tuberculosis. If there is a history of epilepsy treatment with cycloserine should be avoided unless is considered indispensable.

Eighth Cranial Nerve Toxicity

All antituberculosis injectable drugs are toxic to the eight cranial nerve and can cause both vestibular (equilibrium) and cochlear (auditory) damage. It can occur very early in the course of treatment in those patient that received injectables in previous episodes, usually streptomycin which is included in the old WHO Category 2 retreatment regimen. A basal audiometry must be obtained in every patient that will receive as part of the drug regimen a second line injectable. Toxicity is directly related to the accumulated dose and it is irreversible. It's important to ask about tinnitus and/or instability in every monthly visit. If available, audiometry should be carried out every 1-2 months. Hearing loss *may progress even after stopping the injectable drug* and if any hearing loss is detected more frequent hearing testing are warranted. If auditory toxicity is present we can change the dose to 2-3 times per week. If vestibular toxicity is present injectable must be stopped immediately because it will evolve into irreversible ataxia (and probably vertigo) if continued. Since other drugs can cause instability (cycloserine, ethionamide, fluoroquinolones and linezolid) we should try to determine if one of them could be causing the equilibrium disorder before stopping the injectable. ***Remember: auditory and/or vestibular toxicity is irreversible***. In some patients with very extensive disease and complex drug resistance pattern, it will virtually be impossible to stop the injectable prematurely and some auditory toxicity will be unavoidable.

OPHTHALMIC TOXICITY

Optic (retrobulbar) neuritis is mainly caused by ethambutol, due to optic nerve damage. In drug resistant cases the higher doses of ethambutol (25 mg/kg) are frequently used for up to 24 months, increasing the risk of toxicity. Other drugs that might cause ophthalmic toxicity include ethionamide, clofazimine, rifabutin and linezolid. Up to 17% of the patients receiving linezolid will develop severe optic neuritis, especially those patients receiving ≥600 mg daily [6]. When these drugs are going to be used a careful ophthalmologic evaluation must be carried at the start of the regimen and at every monthly visit including visual acuity with a Snellen chart and color discrimination ability with the Ishihara color vision tests.

Rifabutin can cause pan-uveitis characterized by blurry vision, erythema and pain.

GASTROINTESTINAL TOXICITY

Is usually the first to appear after the start of treatment, with nausea and vomiting being the most common; occasionally patients refer abdominal pain. Ethionamide can cause intolerable nausea and vomiting; it also produces a metallic taste in the mouth (dysgeusia) that can cause anorexia and aggravate weight loss and malnutrition.

PAS is without a doubt the antituberculosis drug that causes more gastrointestinal intolerance, with nausea, vomiting and diarrhea that frequently requires discontinuing the drug. Fractioning the daily dose in two can increase tolerance. Monthly liver function tests must be obtained routinely in patients receiving PAS. An antiemetic drug (chloropromazine hydrochloride, ondansetron, domperidone) must be frequently added to control nausea and vomiting; it should be administered at least 30 minutes before the dose of PAS. Proton pump inhibitors (such as omeprazole) or antacids must not be administered within two hours before and after of the drug regimen because they can affect absorption of fluoroquinolones. Patient can eat some toast or crackers before the PAS dose. Despite all these precautions often times PAS must be discontinued due to side effects/toxicity and substituted by other drug if available.

Hepatotoxicity

Hepatic toxicity is the most common adverse effect of antituberculosis treatment and its severity can range from asymptomatic elevation of liver enzymes to fulminant liver insufficiency with encephalopathy and high mortality. Although any patient under treatment with antituberculosis drugs can develop hepatic toxicity, patients with previous liver damage are at higher risk of this complication [7].

Drug related hepatitis can produce virtually any gastrointestinal symptom (nausea, vomiting, abdominal pain, *etc.*). Differential diagnosis should include viral hepatitis, hepatitis A (especially in children) and hepatitis B and C in intravenous drug users (although test for these infections should have been carried out before starting the treatment.

Hepatitis during treatment with first line drugs is more frequently caused by isoniazid, although pyrazinamide is more toxic and produces more severe damage, especially when used at high doses (>30 mg/kg). Rifampin is rarely toxic by itself but can potentiate the toxic effect of isoniazid and pyrazinamide.

If a patient under antituberculosis treatment develops symptoms suggestive of hepatitis, ***all drugs must be stopped immediately*** while waiting for the liver function tests.

Alanine transaminase (ALT) is a better indicator of drug hepatocellular damage than aspartase transaminase (AST), more suggestive of alcohol related damage. An asymptomatic elevation of liver enzymes between 3 to 5 times the upper normal limit does not require modification of treatment regimen, but liver function tests must be monitored weekly. Conversely, in the presence of jaundice, even if liver enzymes are only slightly elevated, treatment should be stopped immediately. If liver enzymes are elevated >5 times the upper normal limit, even if patient is asymptomatic, treatment must be discontinued due to risk of progression to acute liver failure. Hospitalization might be necessary in severe cases.

Once the liver enzymes drop below 2 times the upper normal limit treatment can be restarted. If the availability of non-hepatotoxic drugs allows it, highly toxic drugs like pyrazinamide should not be included in the new regimen. Non-hepatotoxic drugs (injectables, ethambutol, cycloserine) should be started first adding drugs with low hepatotoxic potential (fluoroquinolones). If tolerated, hepatotoxic drugs will then be added to the regimen one at a time while monitoring closely the liver function tests. If the re-introduction of a drug triggers the elevation of liver enzymes, the drug must be stopped and eliminated from the treatment regimen.

ADVERSE HEMATOLOGIC EFFECTS

Practically all antituberculosis drugs can cause hematologic adverse effects including leukopenia, eosinophilia, and neutropenia as well as anemia and thrombocytopenia. These are more frequent in patients receiving linezolid were up to 38% will develop anemia that sometimes will require blood transfusion [6].

HYPOTHYROIDISM

It's a frequent complication in patients under treatment with ethionamide and/or PAS; when these drugs are used simultaneously up to 50% of the patients will develop this side effect. Thyroid function must be monitored at baseline and bimonthly during treatment. When the thyroid stimulant hormone (TSH) level increases to more than two times the upper normal limit, replacement treatment with a daily dose of 50-75 μg of levothyroxine, adjusting the dose based on the results of bimonthly control tests, with a normal value as a target. Most adult patients will require a maintenance dose of 100 μg per day. The adverse effect is reversible once ethionamide and PAS are stopped.

NEPHROTOXICITY

All injectable drugs used in the treatment of MDR-TB are capable of producing renal toxicity [8]. Baseline renal function and monthly monitoring must be carried out in every patient receiving injectable agents, including creatinine clearance in patients with co-morbidities that increase the risk of renal toxicity (*i.e.* patients with diabetes). In patients 60 years or older a lower dose (750 mg per day) is recommended, and if available, serum levels could be used to adjust the dose. If creatinine clearence is <70 mg/ml the injectable can be used three times per week or bi-weekly if <50 mg/ml [9]. If the values of serum creatinine and/or creatinine clearence become abnormal, the injectable must be stopped for a couple of weeks, and depending on the results of renal function tests, determine if treatment can be restarted or definitively discontinued. Since all injectables can cause electrolyte (sodium, chloride, potassium, magnesium, phosphorus and calcium) abnormalities secondary to altered renal clearence, serum levels must be monitored monthly.

MUSCULOSKELETAL ADVERSE EFFECTS

Several antituberculosis drugs, including pyrazinamide, fluoroquinolone, isoniazid, ethionamide and rifabutin can produce myalgia and arthralgia. It is not necessary to stop treatment in most cases.

The incidence of tendon injury associated with fluoroquinolone use is low in healthy individuals, but increases in patients with renal dysfunction; it has been reported with most fluoroquinolones. The median duration of treatment before the onset of tendon injury has been reported as early as 8 days [10]. Elderly patients and those with diabetes are at increased risk. When a patient develops tendinitis the fluoroquinolone should be stopped and treated with non-steroidal anti-inflammatory drugs and rest. In patients with extensive drug resistance, where the fluoroquinolone is a vital part of treatment and its suspension would increase the risk of failure, it might be necessary to continue the drug despite the adverse effect.

CONFLICT OF INTEREST

The author confirms that this chapter has no conflict of interest.

ACKNOWLEDGEMENTS

None declared.

REFERENCES

[1] Curry International Tuberculosis Center and California Department of Public Health. Drug-Resistant Tuberculosis: A Survival Guide for Clinicians. (2nd ed.), 2011.

[2] Farga V, Caminero JA. Tuberculosis. (3rd ed.), Santiago de Chile: Editorial Mediterráneo 2011.

[3] Törün T, Güngör G, Ozmen I, *et al.* Side effects associated with the treatment of multidrug-resistant tuberculosis. Int J Tuberc Lung Dis 2005; 9(12): 1373-7. [PMID: 16468160]

[4] Arbex MA, Varella MdeC, Siqueira HR, Mello FA. Antituberculosis drugs: drug interactions, adverse effects, and use in special situations. Part 2: second line drugs. J Bras Pneumol 2010; 36(5): 641-56. [http://dx.doi.org/10.1590/S1806-37132010000500017] [PMID: 21085831]

[5] Gopal M, Padayatchi N, Metcalfe JZ, O'Donnell MR. Systematic review of clofazimine for the treatment of drug-resistant tuberculosis. Int J Tuberc Lung Dis 2013; 17(8): 1001-7. [http://dx.doi.org/10.5588/ijtld.12.0144] [PMID: 23541151]

[6] Sotgiu G, Centis R, D'Ambrosio L, *et al.* Efficacy, safety and tolerability of linezolid containing regimens in treating MDR-TB and XDR-TB: systematic review and meta-analysis. Eur Respir J 2012; 40(6): 1430-42.
[http://dx.doi.org/10.1183/09031936.00022912] [PMID: 22496332]

[7] Sonika U, Kar P. Tuberculosis and liver disease: management issues. Trop Gastroenterol 2012; 33(2): 102-6.
[http://dx.doi.org/10.7869/tg.2012.25] [PMID: 23025055]

[8] Mingeot-Leclercq MP, Tulkens PM. Aminoglycosides: nephrotoxicity. Antimicrob Agents Chemother 1999; 43(5): 1003-12.
[PMID: 10223907]

[9] Drusano GL, Ambrose PG, Bhavnani SM, Bertino JS, Nafziger AN, Louie A. Back to the future: using aminoglycosides again and how to dose them optimally. Clin Infect Dis 2007; 45(6): 753-60.
[http://dx.doi.org/10.1086/520991] [PMID: 17712761]

[10] Khaliq Y, Zhanel GG. Fluoroquinolone-associated tendinopathy: a critical review of the literature. Clin Infect Dis 2003; 36(11): 1404-10.
[http://dx.doi.org/10.1086/375078] [PMID: 12766835]

CHAPTER 9

Follow Up of Drug Resistant Cases During Treatment

Abstract: This chapter describes the recommended routine for follow-up of drug resistant cases during treatment. Directly observed treatment is absolutely indispensable in patients with drug resistant tuberculosis to avoid the development of further resistance due to inadequate adherence. Monthly evaluation should include active search of side effects and adverse reactions through clinical and laboratory studies. Bacteriological follow-up will consist of monthly sputum smears and cultures, and after culture conversion, monthly sputum smears and bimonthly cultures.

Keywords: Hospitalized, Hemoptysis, Isolation, Monitoring, Out-patient, Promoter, Respiratory distress, Risk.

Strict follow up of any patient being treated for tuberculosis is fundamental for success, but directly observed treatment is absolutely indispensable in patients with drug resistant tuberculosis if one has to avoid the development of further resistance due to inadequate adherence.

FOLLOW-UP OF HOSPITALIZED PATIENTS

Some DR-TB patients will require hospitalization at the start of treatment due to disease complications (respiratory distress, hemoptysis) or to detect and treat early drug side effects. However, unless the hospital has the necessary infrastructure to assure strict respiratory isolation of the patient, health personnel and other patients will be at risk of being infected with a resistant tuberculosis strain. For this reason, the vast majority of drug resistant tuberculosis cases will be treated as outpatients.

OUTPATIENT MONITORING [1, 2]

1. Patients will be supervised daily by the health promoter in charge of directly observed treatment including the administration of the injectable

Rafael Laniado-Laborín

2. By the treating physician at least biweekly during the first month, and once a month thereafter
3. The health promoter must be able to contact the treating physician within 24 hours if the patient develops side or adverse effects
4. During the monthly visit the following items should be actively sought and evaluated:

a. symptoms attributable to tuberculosis
b. side effects and toxicity of drug regimen
c. physical exam including vital signs, body weight, eye examination (Snellen and Ishihara charts)
d. routine safety laboratory tests: blood count, serum chemistry (including renal and liver function tests), urinalysis. Creatinine clearance should be monitored in patients at risk of renal damage (*i.e.* diabetics) receiving injectables
e. bimonthly thyroid function test in patients receiving ethionamide and or PAS
f. monthly audiogram while under injectable treatment
g. monthly sputum smear and culture examination until culture conversion; after culture conversion process smears monthly and culture bimonthly
h. When available, drug serum levels if malabsorption could be an issue (gastrointestinal diseases, lack of clinical/bacteriological response), in small or large patients to assure adequate blood levels or to adjust doses in case of significant side effects

WHEN CAN ISOLATION AND THE USE OF FACEMASKS CAN BE DISCONTINUED IN A PATIENT WITH DRUG RESISTANT TUBERCULOSIS?

Unlike contacts of drug susceptible tuberculosis that can receive preventive treatment with isoniazid for latent tuberculosis infection, there is no treatment with proven efficacy for latent infection in contacts of MDR-TB/XDR-TB cases [3]. One must be especially cautious when deciding to stop isolation (including wearing a facemask). In MDR-TB isolation should be maintained at least until culture conversion.

CONFLICT OF INTEREST

The author confirms that this chapter has no conflict of interest.

ACKNOWLEDGEMENTS

None declared.

REFERENCES

[1] Curry International Tuberculosis Center and California Department of Public Health. Drug Resistant Tuberculosis: A Survival Guide for Clinicians. (2nd ed.), 2011.

[2] Guía para la Atención de Personas con Tuberculosis Resistente a Fármacos. Secretaria de Salud. Primera Edición 2010.

[3] World Health Organization Stop TB Partnership Childhood TB Subgroup. Chapter 4: childhood contact screening and management. Int J Tuberc Lung Dis 2007; 11(1): 12-5. [PMID: 17217124]

CHAPTER 10

Drug Resistant Tuberculosis in Special Situations

Abstract: There are three special situations in drug resistant tuberculosis that merit a more detail description: HIV co-infection, pregnancy and drug resistant TB in children. HIV co-infection: The risk of reactivation of latent tuberculosis infection is 50-100 times higher for subject living with HIV and up to 170 times higher for those with AIDS. Every patient diagnosed with TB must be tested for HIV infection and *vice versa*. The WHO recommends that ARV treatment in patients recently diagnosed as co-infected with HIV and tuberculosis should start within 8 weeks from the start on antituberculosis drugs.

Pregnancy: The best way to deal with MDR-TB during pregnancy is to prevent it. All females of child-bearing age being treated for MDR-TB should be encouraged to adopt an effective contraceptive method or even a combination of them. Most of the drugs used to treat MDR-TB are classified as unsafe during pregnancy or their safety is unknown.

Pediatric tuberculosis: Unlike the adults, most MDR-TB pediatric cases are the result of infection with an already resistant strain, frequently from contact with a household adult. Children with signs and symptoms compatible with active tuberculosis and risk factors for MDR-TB should be started on MDR-TB treatment even if the diagnosis has not been confirmed bacteriologically.

Keywords: Child-bearing, Children, Co-infection, HIV, Pediatric, Pregnancy.

HIV CO-INFECTION

The WHO estimates that 9 million new TB cases and 1.5 deaths were attributed to TB in 2013, and that one third (approximately 2 billion people) of the world population is infected with *M. tuberculosis*. The WHO also estimates that globally, thirty five million people are living with HIV infection and 1.5 million HIV-related deaths occurred in 2013 [1].

The risk for reactivation of latent tuberculosis infection (LTBI) progressing to active TB is 50-110 times higher for patients with HIV co-infection and 110-170

Rafael Laniado-Laborín

times greater for patients living with AIDS. The rate of reactivation of LTBI in immunocompetent individuals (not treated for LTBI) is of 10% for life. The rate of reactivation of LTBI in subjects with HIV infection is approximately 13% *per year* if CD4 cell count is <200, 6% if CD4 count is between 200-350 cells and of 3% if CD4 is >350 cells. Although the number of people dying from HIV-associated TB has decreased since 2004, it was estimated that there were 360 000 deaths from HIV-associated TB in 2013; this corresponds to approximately 25% of all TB deaths [1].

The WHO recommends that every patient with TB should have an HIV test to rule out co-infection (and that every patient seropositive for HIV should be studied to rule out TB. However, less than half of the patients diagnosed with TB worldwide had a documented HIV test result in 2013 [1].

The proportion of HIV patients receiving antiretroviral (ARV) treatment has increased in recent years, currently being at 70%; nonetheless a lot more effort will be needed to reach the ultimate goal of 100% coverage. The proportion of patients with TB co-infected with HIV that are receiving ARV is much lower (less than a third of the patients.

On the other hand, globally only one fifth of the countries globally reported provision of treatment for latent tuberculosis infection in subjects living with HIV in 2013 [1].

TIMING FOR INITIATION OF TREATMENT WITH ARV DRUGS IN PATIENTS CO-INFECTED WITH TB AND HIV

The WHO recommends that ARV treatment in patients recently diagnosed as co-infected with HIV and tuberculosis should start within 8 weeks from the start on antituberculosis drugs [1]. Early initiation of ARV treatment, especially in patients with low CD4+ T-cell counts (<50 per cubic millimeter) increases survival. Deferring the initiation of ARV to the start of the continuation phase of TB treatment (after the first two months) in those with higher CD4+ T-cell counts reduces the risks of Immune Reconstitution Inflammatory Syndrome (IRIS) related to ARV without increasing the risk of AIDS or death [2].

Rifamycins are inducers of cytochrome P-450 and interact with many drugs. Since patients with MDR-TB/XDR-TB are not going to receive rifampin, the interaction of ARV drugs with the TB drug regimen does not represent a problem. Rifampin use will lead to lower level of protease inhibitors and non-nucleoside reverse transcriptase inhibitors [3]. This reduction might be clinically significant in patients over 50 kg (adult patient under 50 kg still get adequate level with standard 600 mg dosing). In adults over 50 kg and on rifampin, expert recommendation is to increase the efavirenz dose to 800 mg total per day. This typically means adding 200 mg of efavirenz to the standard 600 mg. If the efavirenz is in a combo pill (that includes efavirenz, emtricitabine and tenofovir) then just adding 200 mg of efavirenz will be adequate; is important to emphasize that current data is insufficient to support a definitive statement in this regard [4]. While it is true that efavirenz has been extensively used in patients receiving rifampin, in countries with access to many options for ARV treatment drugs without interaction with rifampin could be included in the treatment regimen. Patients that have the co-infection TB-should be treated in collaboration by the TB and HIV programs.

MDR-TB AND PREGNANCY

The best way to deal with MDR-TB during pregnancy is to prevent it. All females of child-bearing age being treated for MDR-TB should be encouraged to adopt an effective contraceptive method or even a combination of them. Most of the drugs used to treat MDR-TB are classified as unsafe during pregnancy or their safety is unknown (Table **10.1**)

Table 10.1. FDA safety classification of medication during pregnancy [5].

A	Adequate and well-controlled studies have failed to demonstrate a risk to the fetus in the first trimester of pregnancy (and there is no evidence of risk in later trimesters).
B	Animal reproduction studies have failed to demonstrate a risk to the fetus and there are no adequate and well-controlled studies in pregnant women
C	Animal reproduction studies have shown an adverse effect on the fetus and there are no adequate and well-controlled studies in humans, but potential benefits may warrant use of the drug in pregnant women despite potential risks

(Table 10.1) contd.....

D	There is positive evidence of human fetal risk based on adverse reaction data from investigational or marketing experience or studies in humans, but potential benefits may warrant use of the drug in pregnant women despite potential risks
X	Studies in animals or humans have demonstrated fetal abnormalities and/or there is positive evidence of human fetal risk based on adverse reaction data from investigational or marketing experience, and the risks involved in use of the drug in pregnant women clearly outweigh potential benefits

According to the FDA classification, besides the drugs in the WHO group 1, none of the other drugs used in treatment of MDR-TB during pregnancy can be classified as an A drug (Table **10.2**)

Table 10.2. Safety of antituberculosis drugs during pregnancy according to the FDA classification.

Ethambutol	**B**
Pyrazinamide	**C**
Kanamycin, Amikacin	**D**
Capreomycin	**C**
Fluoroquinolones	**C**
Ethionamide	**C**
Cycloserine	**C**
PAS	**C**

For this reason, approach to this problem so far has been controversial. Some authors recommend the interruption of pregnancy [6], others recommend suspending treatment completely or limit it to a few drugs [7] and finally, some authors recommend treating pregnant patients with drug regimens similar to non-pregnant patients [8]. Teratogenicity of second line injectables (especially kanamycin and streptomycin) is well documented, causing bilateral eight nerve damage and deafness. By extrapolation amikacin and capreomycin are not recommended, but there are case reports where they have been used safely. Ethionamide has been also associated with congenital defects. Although animal studies have reported congenital malformations in association to fluoroquinolones (arthropathy in puppy models), they have been used in pregnant patients with MDR-TB and there has been no reports of teratogenicity [9].

The largest case series reported so far has been the one from Peru, which included 38 patients [10]. All the patients were treated with individualized regimens that included second line drugs. Although the exact proportion of individual drugs used for treatment was not described in the paper, most of the patients were treated with fluoroquinolones, prothionamide/ethionamide, cycloserine, PAS and either amikacin or kanamycin. In most cases the injectable and ethionamide were suspended or the dose was reduced when pregnancy was diagnosed. At the time of the report (5% were still under treatment) 61% of the patients were discharged as cured, 13% had defaulted, 5% had failed and 13% had died. Five pregnancies ended in spontaneous abortions and one child was stillborn. The authors mention that the rates on the outcome of treatment are the same as that of non-pregnant MDR-TB patients in Peru, and that the obstetric outcomes were similar to those of the general population in the country. Outcomes for the children in the study were good; 12.5% were classified as with low birth weight (<2,500 g) but there were no congenital anomalies in the cohort.

The injectable drugs and ethionamide are considered as teratogens (at least potentially) and should be avoided during the first 6 months of pregnancy. An acceptable (although weak) regimen could include cycloserine, PAS, EMB (if susceptible) and PZA (regardless of the DST results). If the strain has low resistance to INH, high-dose INH could be added to the regimen.

An expert in MDR-TB should be consulted and the risks and benefits of treatments should be discussed with the patient and her family [9].

DRUG RESISTANT TUBERCULOSIS IN CHILDREN

The basic obstacles to understand the epidemiology of drug-resistant tuberculosis in children are the difficulty of confirming the diagnosis, a higher proportion of smear and culture negative cases, a higher frequency of extrapulmonary cases and the low priority assigned to this population segment by tuberculosis programs [11].

According to a recent systematic review, globally, almost 1 million children developed tuberculosis in 2010, and 32,000 of them had MDR-TB [12].

Unlike the adults, most MDR-TB pediatric cases are the result of infection with an already resistant strain, frequently from contact with a household adult (primary resistance) [9].

Risks factors for MDR-TB in children include household contact with a known MDR-TB case or contact with a subject that has failed TB treatment. Due to the difficulty of obtaining an adequate sample for culture and drug susceptibility testing (DST), the diagnosis of MDR-TB in children is usually based on a combination of clinical, radiological and epidemiological data (contact with a known MDR-TB case).

Nonetheless, every effort should be made to obtain bacteriological proof through cultures and DST from sputum, gastric aspirates, lymph node fine needle aspiration and even tissue biopsies. Older children can sometimes produce sputum by induction with hypertonic nebulized saline. In very young children with pulmonary TB, gastric aspirates sometimes will yield positive cultures; bronchoalveolar lavage (BAL) specimens have even lower sensitivity than gastric aspirates samples. If pursued exhaustingly, the diagnosis can be confirmed bacteriologically in more than 50% of the cases.

The availability of molecular based techniques such as the GenoType MTBDRplus (Hain Lifescience, Nehren,Germany) line probe assay and the Xpert MTB/RIF (Xpert; Cepheid, Sunnyvale, California,USA) can provide microbiological diagnosis and DST for rifampin (Xpert) and both rifampin and isoniazid (GenoType MTBDRplus) in a matter of hours instead of months (see Chapter five for more information). The sensitivity of Xpert is approximately 60% for smear-negative culture-positive specimens, which is the most common scenario in children; however its specificity is excellent and thc assay could provide confirmation of the diagnosis and possibly of resistance to rifampin in just a couple of hours. It is important to point out that isolates detected as rifampin resistant with the Xpert might be MDR or mono or polyresistant to rifampin. Clinical practice has shown that up to 80% of strains resistant to rifampin will also be resistant to isoniazid, *i.e.* MDR.

Children with signs and symptoms compatible with active tuberculosis and risk factors for MDR-TB should be started on MDR-TB treatment even if the diagnosis has not been confirmed bacteriologically.

TREATMENT OF DRUG RESISTANT TUBERCULOSIS IN CHILDREN

1. Isoniazid (H) mono-resistance: six months of rifampin (R), pyrazinamide (Z), and ethambutol (E). Patients with extensive disease or slow clinical response might need 9-12 months of treatment.
2. Pirazinamide (Z) mono-resistance: it might be caused by *M. bovis*. Although interhuman transmission of *M. bovis* has been reported [13], most cases are the consequence of the ingestion of unpasteurized milk products. Treatment for Z mono-resistance consists of two months of R-H-E followed by at least 7 months of H and R.

The algorithm for building a treatment regimen in a child with suspected (or proven) MDR-TB is the same as in the adult. The main difference lies in the fact that in most cases the regimen will be empirical and based on the DST of the source case. Some countries will utilize an individualized regimen and other will use a standardized regimen. Drugs for the regimen are selected as follow:

1. Include first line drugs that still retain efficacy according to the source case DST's. PZA will be included regardless of the results of the DST. High dose H could be used if low grade resistance is proven by DST, unless katG mutation is reported
2. Choose an injectable drug. Amikacin is preferred over kanamycin since it has a lower MIC, while capreomycin is usually reserved for XDR-TB cases
3. Select a fluoroquinolone
4. Select as many group four (cycloserine, ethionamide, PAS) drugs as needed to complete a 4-5 drug regimen

As in adults, treatment must be strictly supervised (DOT) and will continue for at least 18-24 months or 18 months after culture conversion (if available)

It is important to point out that pharmacokinetics of antituberculosis drugs in children are different than that of the adults, especially in young children, that usually require a higher dose based on mg/kg of bodyweight to achieve the same pharmacokinetics as adults. One significant practical problem is that second line drugs are seldom available in pediatric formulations requiring splitting or crushing of the tablets leading to inaccurate dosing (either sub or supratherapeutic). Most antituberculosis drugs are not produced in child-friendly formulations and those that are by adding flavor usually have a terrible taste.

Children tend to tolerate adverse effects from second line drugs at lot better than adults [9].

TREATMENT OF PEDIATRIC CONTACTS OF MDR-TB CASES

Pediatric contacts of drug-resistant cases have as high a risk of being infected as the contacts of drug susceptible TB cases [14].

Although there are reports in the literature of treating latent infection in pediatric contacts of MDR-TB cases with different drugs (*i.e.* fluoroquinolones, ethambutol, pyrazinamide) [9], there is no evidence that any of these regimens is effective and/or safe.

A recent systematic review that included over 2,400 references, after excluding papers for different methodological limitations, could not find a single report that recommended an evidence based strategy for treatment of latent TB infection among contacts of MDR-TB [15]. The conclusion of the authors was that the evidence available is not enough (and the existent one is of very low quality) to recommend or reject treatment for latent infection. Our policy in the TB Clinic is to refer pediatric contacts of MDR-TB cases to the Pediatric TB Clinic for a thorough evaluation with the purpose of ruling out active disease, and then monitor the contacts closely for at least two years without treatment.

CONFLICT OF INTEREST

The author confirms that this chapter has no conflict of interest.

ACKNOWLEDGEMENTS

None declared.

REFERENCES

[1] Global tuberculosis report. World Health Organization 2014. ISBN 9789241564809

[2] Abdool Karim SS, Naidoo K, Grobler A, *et al.* Integration of antiretroviral therapy with tuberculosis treatment. N Engl J Med 2011; 365(16): 1492-501. [http://dx.doi.org/10.1056/NEJMoa1014181] [PMID: 22010915]

[3] Ngaimisi E, Mugusi S, Minzi O, *et al.* Effect of rifampicin and CYP2B6 genotype on long-term efavirenz autoinduction and plasma exposure in HIV patients with or without tuberculosis. Clin Pharmacol Ther 2011; 90(3): 406-13.

[http://dx.doi.org/10.1038/clpt.2011.129] [PMID: 21814190]

[4] CDC. Managing Drug Interactions in the Treatment of HIV-Related Tuberculosis. Available from URL: http://www.cdc.gov/tb/TB_HIV_Drugs/default.htm 2013. [online]

[5] Koren G, Pastuszak A, Ito S. Drugs in pregnancy. N Engl J Med 1998; 338(16): 1128-37. [http://dx.doi.org/10.1056/NEJM199804163381607] [PMID: 9545362]

[6] Craig GM, Booth H, Story A, *et al.* The impact of social factors on tuberculosis management. J Adv Nurs 2007; 58(5): 418-24. [http://dx.doi.org/10.1111/j.1365-2648.2007.04257.x] [PMID: 17442025]

[7] Nitta AT, Milligan D. Management of four pregnant women with multidrug-resistant tuberculosis. Clin Infect Dis 1999; 28(6): 1298-304. [http://dx.doi.org/10.1086/514795] [PMID: 10451170]

[8] Shin S, Guerra D, Rich M, *et al.* Treatment of multidrug-resistant tuberculosis during pregnancy: a report of 7 cases. Clin Infect Dis 2003; 36(8): 996-1003. [http://dx.doi.org/10.1086/374225] [PMID: 12684912]

[9] Curry International Tuberculosis Center and California Department of Public Health. Drug-Resistant Tuberculosis: A Survival Guide for Clinicians. (2nd ed.), 2011.

[10] Palacios E, Dallman R, Muñoz M, *et al.* Drug-resistant tuberculosis and pregnancy: treatment outcomes of 38 cases in Lima, Peru. Clin Infect Dis 2009; 48(10): 1413-9. [http://dx.doi.org/10.1086/598191] [PMID: 19361302]

[11] Jenkins HE, Tolman AW, Yuen CM, *et al.* Incidence of multidrug-resistant tuberculosis disease in children: systematic review and global estimates. Lancet 2014; 383(9928): 1572-9. [http://dx.doi.org/10.1016/S0140-6736(14)60195-1] [PMID: 24671080]

[12] Poorana Ganga Devi NP, Swaminathan S. Drug-resistant tuberculosis: pediatric guidelines. Curr Infect Dis Rep 2013; 15(5): 356-63. [http://dx.doi.org/10.1007/s11908-013-0363-z] [PMID: 23990343]

[13] Laniado-Laborín R, Muñiz-Salazar R, García-Ortiz RA, Vargas-Ojeda AC, Villa-Rosas C, Oceguera-Palao L. Molecular characterization of *Mycobacterium bovis* isolates from patients with tuberculosis in Baja California, Mexico. Infect Genet Evol 2014; 27: 1-5. [http://dx.doi.org/10.1016/j.meegid.2014.06.020] [PMID: 24997332]

[14] Laniado-Laborín R, Cazares-Adame R, Volker-Soberanes ML, *et al.* Latent tuberculous infection prevalence among paediatric contacts of drug-resistant and drug-susceptible cases. Int J Tuberc Lung Dis 2014; 18(5): 515-9. [http://dx.doi.org/10.5588/ijtld.13.0840] [PMID: 24903785]

[15] van der Werf MJ, Langendam MW, Sandgren A, Manissero D. Lack of evidence to support policy development for management of contacts of multidrug-resistant tuberculosis patients: two systematic reviews. Int J Tuberc Lung Dis 2012; 16(3): 288-96. [http://dx.doi.org/10.5588/ijtld.11.0437] [PMID: 22640442]

CHAPTER 11

Hypothetical Illustrative Cases

Patients' informed consent was granted to utilize images from their case files to develop these hypothetical cases as long the images are used anonymously.

Abstract: This chapter covers the management of actual MDR/XDR patients with a concise discussion of the importance of previous episodes of TB, the diagnostic algorithm and treatment regimen. Cases with adverse reactions to drugs are also discussed as well as patients with co-morbidities.

Keywords: Adverse reactions, Algorithm, Chest x-rays, Co-morbidities, Culture, DST, Drug-susceptibility tests, GeneXpert®, Management, MDR, Previously treated, Second-line drugs, Toxicity, XDR.

CASE #1

23 year-old male referred to the tuberculosis clinic on June 2010. Negative medical history including smoking, alcohol consumption or illicit drugs.

First diagnosis of tuberculosis in 2005 (based only in positive smears results). Receives treatment with first line drugs ($2HZRE/4H_3R_3$) for six months. Under DOT only during the intensive phase of treatment. Discharged as cured (negative sputum smears). Relapses in 2006; positive sputum smears, no culture. Treated with auto administered WHO Category II regimen ($2HRZES/1HRZE/5R_3H_3E_3$). Discharged as cured with negative sputum microscopy. Second relapse in 2009 with positive sputum smears. This time was treated by a private physician with an unsupervised regimen of RIZ for 13 months despite persistent positive sputum. The patient develops right pyopneumothorax and the patient is referred to a public hospital. A chest tube is placed and after 2 weeks without lung re-expansion the tube is replaced by an open pleurotomy (Eloesser) for adequate drainage (**Fig. 11.1**). Serology for HIV infection was non-reactive. Patient was emaciated weighing only 45 kilograms (BMI 13.1).

Sputum and pleural fluid cultures from admission were positive for *M.*

Rafael Laniado-Laborín

tuberculosis complex and resistant to H (at 0.1 μg/mL and 0.4 μg/mL concentrations), R, Z and S; susceptible to E (first line drugs tested with MGIT960®); second line drug DST (BACTEC 460®) reported susceptibility to capreomycin, ethionamide and levofloxacin.

His admission audiometry revealed auditory damage with abnormal levels at high frequencies (hearing threshold at 40 db for 4,000 Hz).

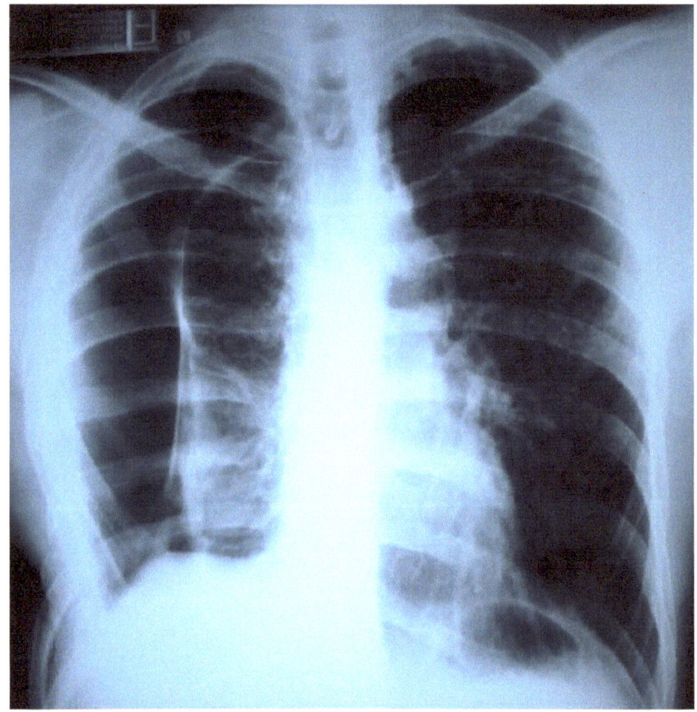

Fig. (11.1). Postoperative chest x-ray with adequate drainage of pus and persistent right pneumothorax and visceral pachypleuritis.

Treatment regimen (started June 2010) included Ethionamide 500 mg QID, Cycloserine 500 mg QID, Levofloxacin (10 mg/kg) 500 mg QID, Ethambutol (25 mg/kg) 1,200 mg QID and Capreomycin (15 mg/kg) 700 mg IM monday through friday. Treatment was directly observed by a health promoter at patient´s home.

The patient converted his sputum cultures after only one month of treatment; the injectable was spaced to three times a week after four months and suspended at six months. Lung collapse required a thoracotomy (at month 16 of treatment) for pleural decortications, which allowed the lung to fully re-expand.

The patient was discharged as cured after 20 months of treatment after culture conversion (April 2012). He is asymptomatic and culture negative after 2 years of follow-up.

Commentary:

1. Although in most developing countries patients are diagnosed just based on sputum microscopy due lack of local access to culture. However patients that fail relapse or are recovered after default MUST have a sputum culture and drug susceptibility testing (DST) to rule out the presence of drug resistant strains. This patient received treatment 3 times without the benefit of DST. It was later proven that in fact the patient was relapsing due to the presence of a drug resistant strain. Most countries will have regional laboratories or at least a national laboratory that can process cultures and DST. Drug resistance could have been detected years earlier avoiding further morbidity (empyema and need for surgery) and transmission of a resistant strain in the community.
2. Patient was treated with the first line retreatment drug regimen that includes the five first line drugs. This goes against a basic tenet of drug resistant TB treatment: never add a single drug to an empirical regimen when re-treating a TB patient. Since 2003 the WHO has recommended that Category II retreatment should be abandoned [1]. In a retrospective cohort of Category I failures patients were either treated with the empirical Category II regimen (if that regimen failed, a standardized regimen including second-line drugs was used) or with a treatment regimen based on DST [2]. Almost 90% of those with DST´s had MDR-TB. Treatment guided by DST´s was 5 times more effective for attaining cure than the Category II regimen (and even three times for effective than those treated with standardized second-line regimen after failure of Category II treatment).
3. HIV must be ruled out in every patient diagnosed with TB (and TB must be ruled out in every patient diagnosed with HIV).
4. Drug susceptibility testing is reliable for H and R of group one drugs and for fluoroquinolones and second line injectables. In this patient, TB strain was resistant to H at both low and medium concentration. This would suggest cross resistance to ethionamide. Even though the DST showed susceptibility to ethionamide the decision was to start treatment with a 5 drug regimen fearing that there might be resistance to ethionamide *in vivo*.

5. Drug regimen was selected as follow: use all drugs from group 1 that DST indicate are still effective. The MGIT results showed that from Group 1, only ethambutol was active against *M. tuberculosis*. However, DST for ethambutol with the MGIT system is unreliable. Since it was reported as susceptible but it was used several times before, a dose of 25 mg/kg was selected. Careful eye exam must be part of the monthly visit to detect early ethambutol optic nerve damage which is usually irreversible. If present ethambutol must be stopped and substituted by another drug if available. It was included in the regimen but not counted as an effective drug. The next step is to select a second line injectable, followed by the selection of a fluoroquinolone. Second line DST showed that the strain was susceptible to capreomycin and levofloxacin. Finally, two drugs were selected from Group 4 (ethionamide and cycloserine) to complete a 4 drug regimen (plus ethambutol). PAS is only used, due to its many side effects, when there is no other option.
6. Audiometry is an integral part of the monthly evaluation. This patient had auditory nerve damage at baseline (maybe related to the use of SM as part of the Category II regimen). Due to his early culture conversion it was possible to space the injectable to 3 times per week at month 4 (after 2 negative cultures) and suspend it after 6 months of treatment. No further damage was observed in follow-up audiometry testing.
7. Some patients will require some type of surgical treatment in this case it was for treatment of pachypleuritis to allow the lung to re-expand. It was decided to perform the surgery well after the patient had converted his cultures and extend treatment for a few months just to be sure to cover a potential bacteremia episode during surgery.
8. Although not evidence based, current recommendation for treatment discharge as cured is at least 18 months of treatment after definitive culture conversion.
9. It is necessary to emphasize the importance of DOT under a personalized health promoter. Treatment of MDR-TB is long (18-24 months), requires the administration of more than a hundred IM injections and patients have to endure many side effects and sometimes toxicities from the drugs. The daily presence of the health promoter gives the patient direct access to the health system and helps in resolving any issues that arise during treatment as soon as they appear.

CASE #2

73 year-old male, peasant for more than 50 years; travels frequently from his village to another state to visit his family abandoning his TB treatment every time he travels. Diagnosed with hypertension (under treatment with captopril) as well as type II diabetes (treatment with glibenclamide/metformin). Never smoked, but

consumed alcohol heavily until 7 years ago. No illicit drug use.

Diagnosed with pulmonary tuberculosis (PTB) in November 2008 treated with first line drugs, unsupervised; abandoned treatment after only two months due to his going back home. Relapsed in March 2010; started treatment in his hometown but abandoned after 4 months when he traveled to another state to visit his family. In January 2012, without the benefit of sputum culture was started on Category II regimen, but abandoned after only two months of treatment.

Referred to the TB Clinic in November 2012; patient was malnourished (44 kg, BMI 17.6). The sputum culture was positive for *M. tuberculosis* complex with resistance to the 5 first line drugs (IRZES). Second line DST showed the strain was susceptible to amikacin, moxifloxacin, capreomycin and ethionamide. His baseline audiometry showed severe auditory impairment; there were extensive lesions in the right upper lobe with large cavities and mediastinal retraction (Fig. **11.2**)

It was decide to treat him with a regimen that included prothionamide 500 mgs QID, cycloserine 500 mgs QID, amikacin 600 mgs IM QID (Monday through Friday), levofloxacin 500 mg QID, PAS 8 grams QID (divided in two doses) and B6 100 mgs QID under DOT by a health promoter at patient´s home.

After only two weeks of treatment the patient presented a severe psychotic episode with visual hallucinations. Cycloserine was stopped immediately. During his monthly visit at the clinic the patient complained of pyrosis, nausea, vomiting and diarrhea. Meclizine, omeprazole and bismuth subsalicylate were added to treatment. Despite the ancillary drugs vomiting becomes incontrollable. PAS was suspended after only 2 months of treatment. Digestive side effects disappeared as soon as PAS was stopped. The patient is left with a three drug regimen only consistent of prothionamide, levofloxacin and capreomycin. Cycloserine was reintroduced at a dose of 250 mg QID and after a couple of weeks increased to 500 mg QID divided in two doses.

His monthly audiometry shows progression of his auditory impairment and it was necessary to suspend capreomycin after only 4 months of sputum conversion.

The patient has tolerated the cycloserine, and currently is asymptomatic after 17 months of treatment and 14 months of sputum conversion.

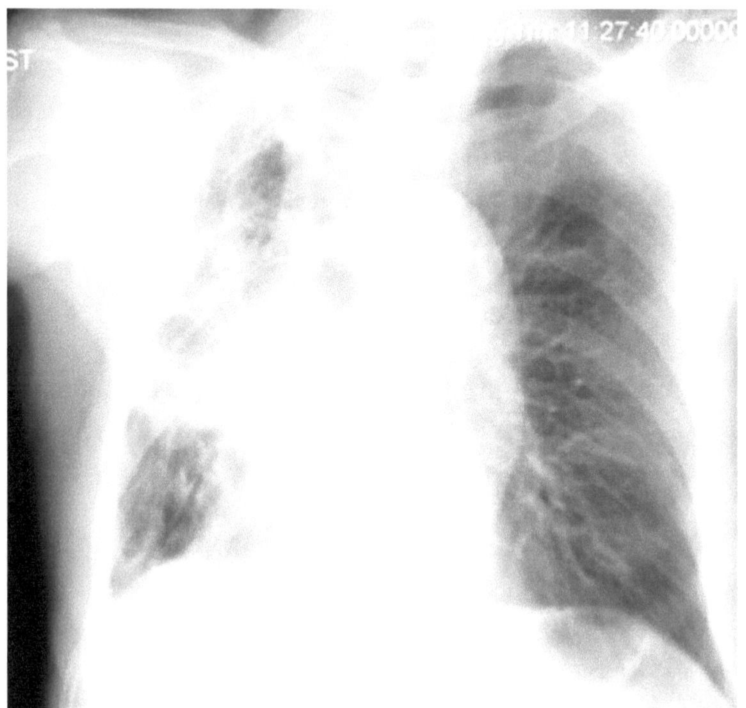

Fig. (11.2). Chest film of patient #2 showing extensive disease.

Commentary:

1. All drugs can have side effects or toxicity, but this is especially true for second line antituberculosis drugs. Several antituberculosis drugs can cause psychotic crisis including cycloserine, fluoroquinolones and isoniazid, although most of the cases are related to cycloserine [3]. The recommendation is to stop cycloserine immediately. Hallucinations stopped after the drug was discontinued. the patient was left with a 4 drug regimen that is still would be classified as appropriate, but one of the drugs is really weak (PAS), so its regimen must be considered as suboptimal with only three potent drugs.
2. The patient then develops intolerable digestive side effects that not respond to ancillary treatment and we are forced to stop PAS. At this juncture the decision to restart cycloserine was taken despite the history of central nervous system toxicity. An initial dose of 250 mgs QID for two weeks followed by 250 mgs BID was well tolerated without neurologic side effects.

3. After 4 months of culture conversion it was necessary to stop the injectable due to progressive hearing loss. This could be appropriate for a patient left with a strong oral regimen, but this patient was left with a three drug regimen of which only two are considered as potent (fluoroquinolone and injectable). The possibility of adding linezolid was contemplated but due to its high cost it was unavailable. The value of drugs from group five besides linezolid has been proven to be questionable [4]. The patient is currently in his last month of treatment after 17 months of culture conversion.
4. When treating an older patient, even without co-morbidity, one must be aware that the threshold for side effects/toxicity might be lower and must be very careful in monitoring renal function.

CASE #3

53 year-old male. Heavy smoker (40 pack-years) and intense alcohol consumption; drug user for more than 30 years including IV heroin. Patient was diagnosed with pulmonary tuberculosis (sputum smear 3+; Fig. **11.3**); sputum culture was positive for *M. tuberculosis*, susceptible to all first line drugs).

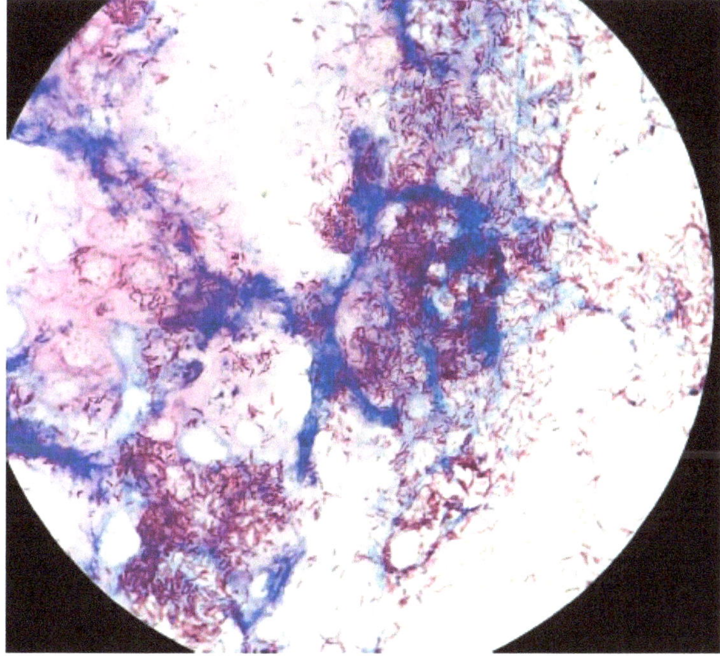

Fig. (11.3). Sputum smear AFB positive (3+).

The chest film shows extensive bilateral disease, with cavities in both upper lobes and airspace densities in virtually all the rest of the lung fields (Fig. **11.4**).

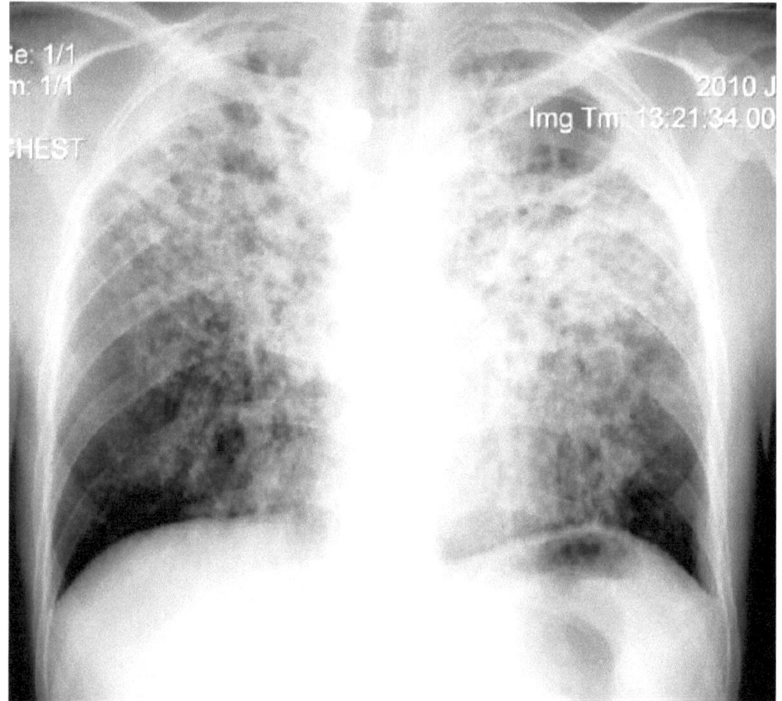

Fig. (11.4). Chest film with extensive bilateral disease.

Starts treatment and after two months develops clinical hepatitis with jaundice (initial AST 39 IU, ALT 29 IU; after two months AST rose to 722 IU and ALT to 578 IU, total bilirubin 17.8 mg/dL). His liver ultrasound reveals a small nodular liver (suggestive of cirrhosis), splenomegaly and ascites. Viral panel was non reactive for HIV and hepatitis B, but reactive for hepatitis C. Treatment is suspended and in approximately one month the liver enzymes have decreased to AST 133 IU and ALT to 107 IU and bilirubin to 6.4 mg/dL. The patient was very symptomatic with high fever, productive cough, dyspnea and weight loss. A modified regimen including second line drugs was started with levofloxacin 750 mg QID (64 kg BMI 22.4), rifampin 600 mg QID, ethambutol 1,200 mg QID and amikacin 1 g IM QID (Monday through Friday). One week later the patient liver function tests show AST 348 IU and ALT 252 IU. Rifampin is stopped and cycloserine is started at 250 mg BID. One week later the ALT is reported at 161 IU. One month later the patient is afebrile, and the symptoms attributable to pulmonary TB have subsided. Liver function test are reported with AST 123 IU, ALT 105 IU and bilirubin 1.89 mg/dL.

Commentary:

1. Co-morbidities will complicate (even more) the treatment of MDR-TB. The threshold for many side effects will be lower in patients with renal or hepatic disease and patients with diabetes, due to retinopathy and nephropathy, will frequently require a modification of treatment regimen, a difficult situation since there are usually not many other drug options. This patient had liver cirrhosis due to hepatitis C, and quickly developed hepatic failure while under treatment with first line drugs [5]. The more hepatotoxic of the first line drugs is pyrazinamide, and in case of drug induced hepatitis it should be stopped immediately and never used again. Isoniazid and rifampin (to a much lesser degree) can also cause liver damage. It was necessary to start treatment for TB since the patient was deteriorating. After the liver function tests showed enough improvement a modified regimen including second line drugs was started, including rifampin; however, after only a week it was necessary to stop rifampin due to an increase of the liver enzymes. It was substituted with another second line drug, cycloserine. At the end a patient with a pan-susceptible infection needed a regimen that included three second line drugs.
2. Patients with co-morbidities will require close clinical and laboratory monitoring for early detection of adverse effects. It may be necessary also to adjust the dose of certain drugs depending on the type of co-morbidity. For example, in the presence of renal failure some drugs (please refer to Chapter 6) will require adjustment and spacing of the doses.
3. Sometimes it is not possible to wait for a complete normalization of the laboratory tests due to rapid progression of tuberculosis; this patient had extensive disease and was rapidly deteriorating. It must be decided in cases like these the risk/benefit ratio of restarting treatment instead of waiting without it.

CASE #4

33 year-old female, housewife; no significant medical history. She was treated 2 years ago for pulmonary TB. Diagnosis was based only on sputum smears. Treatment with first line drugs ($2HRZE/4R_3H_3$) was not directly observed. She was discharged as cured after 6 months of treatment. The patient relapses six

months ago with symptoms and positive sputum smears. She is started on unsupervised treatment again with the same regimen; she defaulted after three months when she was receiving the first month of the follow-up phase ($4R_3H_3$). She seeks medical attention due to reappearance of symptoms. Her sputum smears are reported as positive 3+. There are several options for managing this patient:

a. Should treatment with first line drugs be reinitiated from the start?
b. Should treatment with first line drugs be reinitiated from where she defaulted?
c. Should a sputum sample be obtained for culture and first and second line DST and wait for the results to start treatment?
d. Should we start an empirical standardized regimen with second line drugs and obtain a sample for culture and DST?

Commentary:

1. Although the empirical use of first line drugs for a third time is not considered a good option due to the high risk of increasing the degree of potential undetected drug resistance, the correct answer depends on your resources. Ideally, a molecular technique for rapid diagnosis of resistance (GeneXpert® and/or Genotype MTBDRplus® should be carried out when the case is recovered. A patient with resistance to R ("pre-MDR") or resistance to H & R (MDR) obviously should not be treated with the primary regimen. If the patient is proven to be MDR she should be started on a standardized second line regimen. If MGIT or MODS are available we could have the results for the rest of the first line drugs within 1-3 weeks and then modify the regimen if necessary. The history in this case reveals that she only received first line drugs, consequently the probability of resistance to second line drugs will depend on the prevalence of drug resistance rates for second line drugs in the region. There are regions in the world were unfortunately, rates of resistance to fluoroquinolones and second line injectable are already high, increasing the risk of acquiring a resistant strain in the community. The initial sputum sample should subsequently be tested for second line drug susceptibility, at least for fluoroquinolones and second line injectables.
2. If the samples must be sent to a central laboratory (or to a supranational laboratory) the result might be available only after a few months. During this period the patient will deteriorate and will be transmitting a potentially resistant strain generating new cases. Although a high proportion of relapses in patients whose regimen included rifampin for the whole course and were under ***directly observed treatment*** are usually due to pan-susceptible MTB strains, this patient was not supervised during either of her two

treatments, increasing the risk of current drug resistance. Cases like this highlight the urgent need to expand the availability of test for rapid diagnosis of tuberculosis and resistance to first line drugs, and also the need to strengthen local and regional tuberculosis laboratories to increase their ability to conduct cultures and DST and decrease the need to centralize these services.

CASE #5

20 year-old male is referred to the TB Clinic. He has a history of being diagnosed with PTB as a new case, based only on clinical features and positive sputum smears. Despite lack of sputum conversion after four months of primary regimen (daily RHZE) he was started on the intermittent phase (HR three times per week). He was symptomatic (productive cough, fever) and his chest x-ray show extensive destruction of the left lung (Fig. **11.5**).

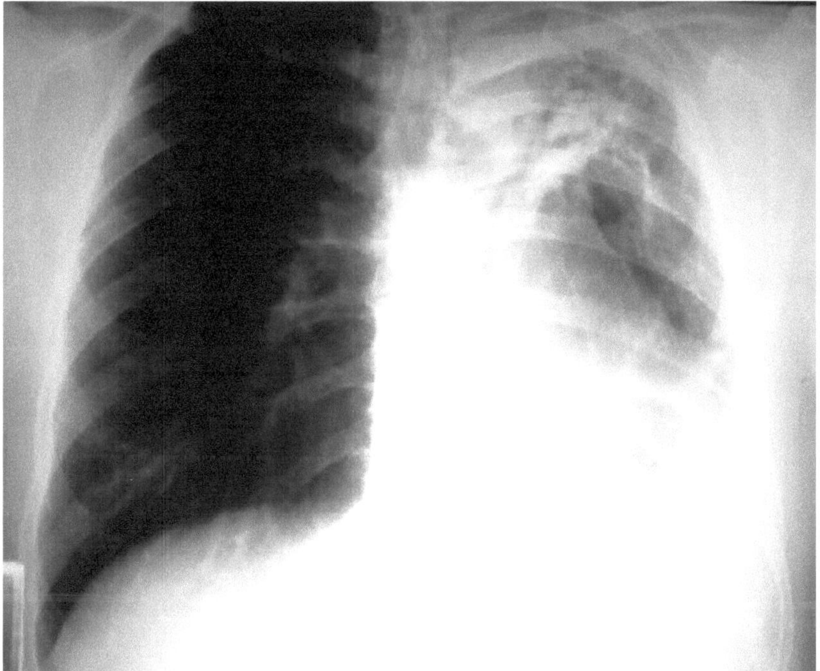

Fig. (11.5). Chest x-ray film showing extensive destruction of left lung with mediastinal and diaphragmatic retraction.

His sputum culture confirmed the presence of *M. tuberculosis* resistant to H, R, E & S. The strain in the same sample was reported resistant to Z in on laboratory and resistant in another (both tested with the MGIT 960® system); low grade resistance (0.25 µg) to moxifloxacin was reported from second line drugs. The strain was susceptible to ethionamide, capreomycin and amikacin.

Patient starts treatment with Prothionamide (500 mg), Cycloserine (500 mg), Moxifloxacin (400 mg), Amikacin (1 g) and PAS (8g) under home DOT supervised by a health promotor. Converts culture in three months. The injectable was stopped after 4 consecutive negative monthly cultures.

After 9 months of consecutive cultures a Lowenstein Jensen culture showed growth of *M. tuberculosis* and it was decided to stop treatment and get new DST including for second line drugs. The strain is resistant to H (both at 0.1 and 0.4 µg/mL), R, E, S and moxifloxacin (pyrosequencing showed mutations 91 CCG & 90 GTG that are associated to low grade resistance to moxifloxacin. It was susceptible to ethionamide, pyrazinamide, capreomycin and amikacin.

A new treatment regimen includes levofloxacin (750 mg), cycloserine (500 mg), prothionamide (500 mg), capreomycin (1 g), linezolid (600 mg) and Z (1,500 mg). 100 mg of B6 were added to the regimen. Culture becomes negative after 4 months of treatment.

A lung perfusion gammagram showed that the left lung has virtually no perfusion (Fig. **11.6**).

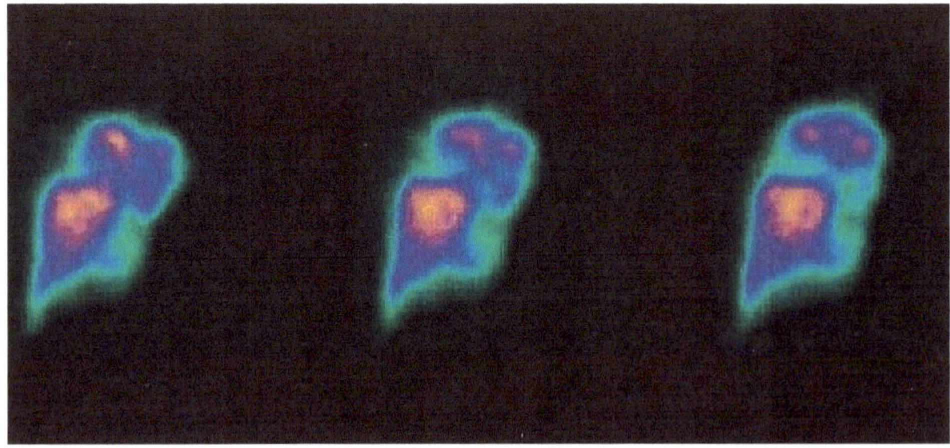

Fig. (11.6). Lung perfusion gammagram showing almost complete lack of perfusion in left lung.

Commentary:

1. It is highly likely that this patient was infected with a resistant strain as a new case; that would explain why he failed treatment with first line drugs and never converted to sputum negative. This could have prevented if DST have been carried out with a rapid test (GeneXpert®, Genotype®, MODS) at the time of initial diagnosis, and even with an automated liquid culture system (*e.g.* MGIT 960®) that would render results before a month. Resistance would have been timely detected and the patient would have been treated with an effective regimen preventing further development of drug resistance. Regions with high burden of drug resistant cases *must* culture *all* new cases.
2. DST for second line drugs is reliable only for fluoroquinolones (levofloxacin and moxifloxacin) and injectables (amikacin, kanamycin and capreomycin). The fact that the strain was resistant to low concentration of H suggests that it would also be resistant to ethionamide (since this is related to the same gene mutation). However phenotypic testing in this case reported susceptibility to ethionamide.
3. Despite being treated with an adequate regimen under strict DOT the patient failed eventually. The new DST was virtually identical to the original, and thus failure was not attributable to extended resistance. A perfusion gammagram shows that the left lung virtually have no blood circulation and consequently the amount of drug reaching left lung tissue would be almost nil. Administration of inhaled aminoglycosides has been reported for treating mycobacteria [6]. This patient must be evaluated by a thoracic surgeon to determine if a left pneumonectomy is feasible. If the left lung is not removed there is a high risk of failure to drug treatment.

CONFLICT OF INTEREST

The author confirms that this chapter has no conflict of interest.

ACKNOWLEDGEMENTS

None declared.

REFERENCES

[1] Espinal MA. Time to abandon the standard retreatment regimen with first-line drugs for failures of standard treatment. Int J Tuberc Lung Dis 2003; 7(7): 607-8. [Editorial].
[PMID: 12870678]

[2] Saravia JC, Appleton SC, Rich ML, Sarria M, Bayona J, Becerra MC. Retreatment management strategies when first-line tuberculosis therapy fails. Int J Tuberc Lung Dis 2005; 9(4): 421-9.
[PMID: 15830748]

[3] Törün T, Güngör G, Özmen I, *et al.* Side effects associated with the treatment of multidrug-resistant tuberculosis. Int J Tuberc Lung Dis 2005; 9(12): 1373-7.
[PMID: 16468160]

[4] Chang KC, Yew WW, Tam CM, Leung CC. WHO group 5 drugs and difficult multidrug-resistant tuberculosis: a systematic review with cohort analysis and meta-analysis. Antimicrob Agents Chemother 2013; 57(9): 4097-104.
[http://dx.doi.org/10.1128/AAC.00120-13] [PMID: 23774431]

[5] Arbex MA, Varella M de C, Siqueira HR, Mello FA. Antituberculosis drugs: drug interactions, adverse effects, and use in special situations. Part 1: first-line drugs. J Bras Pneumol 2010; 36(5): 626-40.
[http://dx.doi.org/10.1590/S1806-37132010000500016] [PMID: 21085830]

[6] Davis KK, Kao PN, Jacobs SS, Ruoss SJ. Aerosolized amikacin for treatment of pulmonary *Mycobacterium avium* infections: an observational case series. BMC Pulm Med 2007; 7: 2.
[http://dx.doi.org/10.1186/1471-2466-7-2] [PMID: 17319962]

SUBJECT INDEX

Rafael Laniado-Laborín

www.ingramcontent.com/pod-product-compliance
Lightning Source LLC
Chambersburg PA
CBHW041717210326
41598CB00007B/690
9781681080673